Life and Leisure for the Physically Handicapped

Life and Leisure for the Physically Handicapped

Ruth Elliott

Elek Books Limited
2 All Saints Street London N1

Life & Leisure

Published by
ELEK BOOKS LIMITED
2 All Saints Street London N1

ISBN 0 236.17661.7

Made and printed in Great Britain by
Weatherbys Printers
Wellingborough Northants

Contents

List of illustrations

Introduction

A physical handicap is something that can happen to anybody, temporarily or permanently, through accident, illness, bad luck, or just sheer genetic cussedness.

It *has* happened to many people in every civilized community. Although the exact figures are still in dispute, it has been estimated that one person in ten is affected by physical disability of one sort or another, either as a sufferer, relative of a sufferer, employer, teacher, social worker, or just well-intentioned friend. The numbers are likely to increase, as more physically handicapped children survive beyond babyhood, more elderly people live to develop physical handicaps at the other end of our lengthening life-span, and more toll is taken by technical progress in the shape of accidents due to transport, complicated machinery in peace and war, competitiveness in sport, youthful enterprise, or just bad luck.

Fortunately, many physically disabled people can continue to lead full, happy and successful lives. To some extent, at least, advances in modern medicine and technology can help them to get about, to replace a missing or defective part of the body, to supplement a faulty faculty.

It can be done, and it has been done. But it is not always seen to be done. Everybody knows about the conspicuous successes: President Roosevelt, Helen Keller, Michael Flanders the actor, Douglas Bader, the legless air ace, Kenneth Horne, making a fighting comeback into the worlds of business and entertainment after a stroke, Jack Ashley, the deaf MP, Lady Masham of Ilton, the wheelchair-bound life peeress, racing drivers Stirling Moss and Graham Hill and probably many others. These physically disabled people are, or have been, in the public eye: their success is enhanced by the extra effort it has cost them.

But there are many more physically disabled people well known because they are successful businessmen, doctors, architects, artists, writers, administrators, and so on, who do not wish to have any allowance made for the fact that they happen also to be physically disabled. It may be a fact which complicates their daily lives, but they have won this daily battle, and do not wish to make capital out of their private struggle.

This attitude may be part of a pre-Freudian, stiff-upper-lip tradition, and cannot always be easy to maintain. It inspires respect, although it runs counter to the modern habit of letting one's hair down, and discussing all sorts of problems in public, in the hope of discovering that one's worst private horror is not unique, and that someone else has already found a solution to it.

Unfortunately, it deprives many other physically handicapped people of the comforting realization that someone, much like themselves, has managed to adapt entirely to a successful personal, professional and domestic life. They may not be able to perform certain physical actions which other people take casually for granted. But physical prowess is not all-important. Sometimes the very inability to diffuse one's energies on the football field, the golf course, or the dance floor, may act as an extra spur, especially to a handicapped child or young person who longs to fit in and excel at something.

Today, physical handicap need no longer be regarded merely as an affliction inspiring, at best, pity. Rather it can be seen as a challenge. Physically handicapped people are no longer labelled 'blind' or 'crippled' and left at that. Many of them can be helped to live nearly normal lives, go to work, get married, travel, enjoy themselves, and help others. Numerous enquiries into their needs have been set afoot. Organizations and societies have been formed by people, often themselves personally concerned with physical handicap, to provide help, information and advice to sufferers from illnesses like multiple sclerosis, diabetes, epilepsy, muscular dystrophy and many others (see list in Appendix).

The most encouraging fact about all the interest now centring on the precise numbers and needs of the physically disabled is the recognition that a great deal can be done to help them live constructively.

Of course suitable housing, education, special facilities are all vitally important to health, comfort, ease of mind. Once these basic necessities have been provided, either privately or by the State, they frequently enable the physically handicapped to take one of a large range of jobs, to support their families and to help other people maybe more handicapped than themselves. They can fulfil themselves as individuals, and contribute to the community as much and as satisfyingly as any able-bodied person.

A blind student training for social work, a polio-disabled housewife running a home for her family from her wheelchair, a paraplegic demonstrating the electronic device which enables him to hold down a job, all are gravitating from the position of recipient of society's care to the credit side of the ledger. An invalid or elderly person who can be helped to live independently is not only relieving the community from looking after him but almost certainly also leading a much happier, personally more satisfying existence.

But for many of the physically handicapped, even ordinary everyday life requires heroic qualities including patience, endurance, courage, persistence and a special brand of determined cheerfulness. Many severely handicapped people demonstrate this only too successfully day after day without self-consciousness or reference to their special problem.

There is, for instance, the legless thalidomide boy in a nursery school whose prowess on his artificial legs is such that all the other children envy him; the blind sociologist who relies on his sighted secretary for his research; the voluble chairbound journalist who writes up the food he consumes during an evidently full and social visiting round of restaurants and hotels; the bed-bound architect whose wife helps him with the facts for the articles he writes for the technical press; the deaf and dumb chairbound church worker who leads an active official life by means of a child's alphabet tablet on which he taps out messages at incredible speed; the athetoid spastic writer whose sole usable limb is his left foot with which he has been taught to type.

Sometimes, their physical handicap has led sufferers to undertake work no one else has thought of doing, like Meg Du Boisson, the energetic and articulate founder of the Disablement

Income Group (see page 119) who suffered from multiple sclerosis but died in fact in a traffic accident on her way to its Annual General Meeting; or Ann Armstrong, editor of *The Responaut*, who publishes her magazine 'by, for and about gadget-aided people' in addition to leading an apparently full life from within the confines of an iron lung; or Mary Greaves, present director of the Disablement Income Group who investigated the whole field of employment of the physically handicapped after a lifetime's work as teacher and civil servant, unhampered by the fact that she herself has been disabled by polio.

In writing this book, I have had in mind principally three categories of the physically disabled and chronically sick:

1. *Children*
   Possibly the group best catered for by existing services providing information and training facilities. These children really merit all the attention and training they can get since many of them may well become fully-integrated members of the community, to their own and everybody else's advantage. Without it, their lives may be prolonged but neither happy nor fulfilled.

2. *The elderly*
   Certainly the largest group, with needs which are widespread, if not always well known. One difficulty here is that many elderly people deteriorate so slowly that it is difficult to pin-point the day when they first find that they can no longer go downstairs or cook a hot meal for themselves, so that medical attention is not always alerted.

3. *All those in between*
   These people often have social and living problems which go beyond the scope of doctors and hospitals. Their standard of living is often below that of comparable families because of the special difficulties many physically disabled people experience in finding work unless they have some special skill or knowledge. Their living accommodation is often less convenient because the lack of, say, hot water, an indoor WC, or a self-contained kitchen, which would inconvenience even an able-bodied person, tends to make their lives nearly impossible. A disabled housewife, too, has personal

and practical domestic problems which will affect her entire family, especially if she has small children. She may not be able to manage the housework, the cooking and the shopping without help. Maybe she can't even do her own hair, dress herself or comfort a sobbing child with a good cuddle.

In writing this book, I have tried to provide as many answers as possible to questions asked by physically disabled people, and by the parents or other people who may be caring for them. But one of the main points I want to make is to persuade people to go out and look for help, to ask questions, contact organizations, especially the British Red Cross Society. Even if the first approaches provide little immediate constructive help, your efforts will snowball. One of the advantages of a modern society served by modern means of communication is that we can all learn from one another. Few problems are unique, and those which have been solved once can probably be solved elsewhere by much the same means.

Chapter 1

'Us' and 'them'

It may sound as glib and soulless as an Act of Parliament to remind a struggling mother of a severely disabled child, or an old lady faced with the horror of losing her sight, that there are sources of help to which she can turn.

Some of these, like a pension or allowance, or the facilities of the National Health Service, are provided by the State at national level; most others come through the local authority. Beyond these are the numerous voluntary organizations, many linked to the local authorities in providing for the physically disabled living at home.

Unfortunately, many people simply don't take advantage of the services which exist for them. In some cases, this may be because it all seems too much trouble or because they can't bring themselves to fill in yet another application form or have another interview with a strange official. After all, what can anyone really do for them? Who can redress the balance of nature?

But, surely, even half a loaf is better than no bread at all; and even though no one can restore a patient to full health or mobility, a wheelchair, for example, or even a specially adapted car, might enable him to go out to work, shop, visit, or become more independent. Another reason why help does not always percolate to the most deserving cases is the sturdy individualism of many physically disabled people: a determination to cope on their own, if they're only allowed to get on with it.

So the health visitor or medical social worker never meets the very people who could most benefit from what she has to offer, and some brave old soul saves up for a wheelchair when one could be provided free, gratis, and for only a recommendation from the GP or hospital consultant. Or the mother of a deaf child does not bring him to the clinic where his trouble could be analyzed and may be already corrected before he starts his schooling because she is half-afraid that other mothers will think him mentally deficient.

But the single most prevalent reason why people don't apply for services, aids, grants, or other help is BECAUSE THEY DON'T REALISE THEY ARE ENTITLED TO THEM.

The Handicapped Persons' Register

Probably not more than one out of every three physically disabled people have themselves included on their local authority's Handicapped Persons' Register. (This is quite a different and separate service from the register kept by the local Labour Exchanges under the Handicapped Persons (Employment) Act which, as its title implies, affects only people of working age who are seeking re-training or a job. See page 99 for this.)

Local authorities vary, and so do the services they provide, but surely nothing is lost, and quite a lot can be gained, by simply putting one's name forward for anything to which one may quite legitimately be entitled in the shape of aids and appliances, home help or a grant or loan towards a home improvement or adaptation, or whatever.

Local authorities for their part would be greatly helped in deciding what sort of services are needed in their areas if more disabled people registered, and could then, in turn, more easily inform the disabled what facilities for them exist.

Application for inclusion in the register should normally be made to the local authority's welfare department, either personally, or through the GP or hospital concerned. It's equally possible to apply personally, or on behalf of an aged parent or even a neighbour who may have no close relatives.

Statutory authorities

It has already been pointed out that services provided by local authorities for the physically disabled vary from one area to another. In some places, laundry services, luncheon clubs, cash grants for home adaptations may be available. In others, there may be home visiting, out-work for the housebound, a mobile library. In a third, the physically disabled may have to rely largely on the efforts of voluntary organizations.

One reason for this discrepancy is that official services for the disabled have, until now, been lodged under different departments variously called 'welfare', 'health', 'education', 'social welfare' or even 'housing'. All this was apt to be confusing to an applicant for a specific service. An alteration in geographical boundaries, or, as in London in 1965, in demarcation of powers between authorities, can bewilder even experienced social workers or GPs as they try to work out who is responsible for what.

Fortunately, there is now the prospect that further statutory changes, like, for instance, the Chronically Sick and Disabled Persons Act, and the recommended reorganization of certain local government departments, will produce some uniformity, not only in the provision of social and medical services but also in nomenclature. Eventually, 'social service' departments will be the ones mainly concerned with physically handicapped people living at home.

Another difficulty is the fact that in the U.K. social services are only partly provided by the local authorities. This is one field where government (local as well as national) often works hand in hand with the numerous voluntary organizations. They became experts in looking after the less fortunate members of the community in the past when only do-gooders or people with a social conscience concerned themselves with such subjects.

Nowadays, governments are expected to involve themselves in all aspects of the lives of the people they govern. Certainly, they are easily blamed if things are not going well. In administering the social services, however, the U.K. compromise has been to make use of the energy, drive and accumulated expertise of the voluntary organizations, and for government agencies to work hand in hand with them in providing facilities like meals-on-wheels, chiropody, transport, swimming tuition, and many others which neither group might have been able to produce unaided. It is partly because so many different or combined sponsors may be involved that it is often difficult to say precisely what social services beyond the statutory minimum are available in various parts of the country. In many areas the local Council for Social Service, acting often in conjunction with the local authority, has compiled a *Directory of Social Services* to act as a guide not only to people in need but even for experienced but often busy social workers and General Practitioners.

Among the kind of services rendered by local authorities either directly or indirectly, are: home nursing, chiropody (at home or in a clinic), home helps, laundry for the very aged and incontinent, loan of special nursing equipment, home aids and adaptations, meals-on-wheels delivered to homes or luncheon clubs which also have a social function, social or work centres for the handicapped, help with holidays and outings, the provision of special schools and housing, industrial rehabilitation, training for work, and the finding of suitable jobs.

Voluntary organizations

Organizations for the under-privileged are not in themselves new. In the past, people with a social conscience and a concern for the under-dog set up charities for the blind, the deaf, the crippled, and these have been joined by newer, maybe brasher and flourishing and useful organizations whose activities have helped generations of sufferers, nationally and locally.

In the last ten to twenty years these established, experienced organizations have been joined by newer, maybe brasher and more publicity-conscious voluntary organizations which are helping to focus public attention on getting visible results. Many of them are concerned with individual illnesses or conditions (muscular dystrophy, multiple sclerosis, epilepsy, cerebral palsy, etc.; see list of names and addresses on pages 130-7). Often they have been started by individual sufferers themselves, by their close relatives, or by others intimately concerned with the day-to-day problems such people were living with. Undoubtedly they have brought many disabled people previously outside the social network into contact with others similarly afflicted, and provided them with new interests, activities and hopes.

If you want a job well done, it's still not enough to do it yourself. Even the most poignant personal involvement cannot in itself replace administrative skill, medical knowledge, and a general appreciation of the economic facts of life. Still, most if not all the voluntary bodies which sprang into vehement and articulate life are now helping to smooth life for many of their hitherto uncategorized members. Many people enjoy the relief of meeting others who share their particular living and working problems, although members who are not inclined to do so need not become personally or socially involved in the organization they have joined for strictly practical purposes.

Unlike social or political clubs, most of the voluntary organizations for specific ailments are not exclusive to sufferers from that ailment. They face too many common problems about living and housing, getting around and about, education and work, and have already made too many strides in the provision of transport, job assessment, holidays, etc. to keep all such facilities jealously to themselves. There is no need to make an agonizing choice between joining, say, the *Spastics Society* or the *National Deaf Children's Society*, even if your cerebrally palsied child cannot hear. The *Spastics Society* in particular will advise all sorts of handicapped people – which is just as well since few of the physically handicapped fit neatly into one slot as an arthritic or a man with one leg. They may also suffer from deafness or chronic asthma or diabetes so that they may wonder whether to address themselves first to the *British Rheumatism and Arthritis Association*, the *Diabetic Association* or the *Royal National Institute for the Deaf*.

But it is not only on the individual, local level of sufferer-to-sufferer that the voluntary organizations have made their mark. In some fields they are well launched into research which no government agency has yet undertaken.

In particular, the *National Fund for Research into Crippling Diseases* is an umbrella organization whose monumental four-volume buying guide, *Equipment for the Disabled* (ed. by Margaret Agerholm which can be seen at large public libraries or ordered from the NFRCD – see Appendix for address – for 7 guineas) is an invaluable help when buying sickroom and other specialized equipment for the disabled. The *Disabled Living Foundation* (same address) is another major source of support in providing information on equipment, dress, alterations in the home, holidays and activities.

Among the more specific societies for one or other group of physically disabled, the employment and social work department of the *Spastics Society* is helpful in finding work for spastics who can be trained for specific jobs, although they modestly point out that their efforts are made very much in conjunction with those of the Department of Employment The *Royal National Institute for the Deaf* publishes a very useful booklet, *Special Aids to Hearing*, which lists not only its valuable hearing aid test service but other aids many deaf people may not even know about: light-flashing alarms, visual doorbells, baby alarms and aids to telephoning and TV-viewing.

The *Royal National Institute for the Blind* sells apparatus, equipment and games direct to blind people through its sales department.

But the organizations of interest to disabled people go beyond those dealing with specific illnesses and conditions. Many concern themselves with the problems of special groups, including house-bound invalids, disabled drivers, the elderly, children with educational difficulties and others (see alphabetical index). Many publish regular magazines and collect information on subjects of interest to their members.

In some areas there is no longer such a sharp delineation between the needs of the able-bodied and those of the physically handicapped. *The Consumers' Association* has investigated invalid tricycles and the affiliated *Research Institute for Consumer Affairs* in conjunction with the *National Fund for Research into Crippling Diseases* has tested products of interest to disabled users, including reading aids, refrigerators, cookers, microfilm projectors, prismatic spectacles and armchairs, with methods similar to those used for evaluating ordinary branded goods in their monthly magazine *Which?* It found, not really all that surprisingly, that many able-bodied people would also prefer household goods to be made in ways which would eliminate awkward stretchings and potentially difficult-to-use switches, and may thus eventually effect generally beneficial results in quite ordinary consumer goods.

Because the physically disabled are just another group in the community in need of help, other voluntary organizations have become concerned with helping them. This includes, for instance, young members of local Church groups, scouts and guides, *Community Service Volunteers*, *Task Force*, *Young Volunteer Force*, etc. who may be willing to shop for a house-bound patient, visit him in his home and decorate it if necessary, organize outings for handicapped children or supervise their sporting activities. The *Women's Royal Voluntary Service* (WRVS) too, *Rotary Clubs*, and the *British Legion* provide occasional help at local level to the physically disabled, not specifically, but as just another of the problems of the community in which they live.

Is our whole society becoming more compassionate? One effect of modern life is certainly that more people get to know about each other and each other's problems. But one official admitted to her amazement on finding that voluntary work is by no means only a one-way traffic. 'Our members really thrive on helping others,' she said. 'It brings them out of their shells – makes them feel that their lives are really worth living to someone besides themselves.'

Chapter 2

Living at home

It is generally accepted – especially maybe by people living in convenient modern homes – that even a bad home is better than living in a good institution. But, of course, a good home, or one which has been specially improved to suit the individual needs of its occupant, is better still.

Too many able-bodied people treat the physically handicapped as though he were also likely to be feeble-minded. They talk round him instead of to him and arrange his outings and his affairs as though he were a child. Sometimes they even take it upon themselves to tell him how and where to live, what clothes to wear or what foods to eat.

This attitude is not only ridiculous (since it implies that someone who can't, for instance, do up his shoelaces or dial a telephone because he has lost the use of his hand must also in other respects be as dependent as the child of four he resembles in this way only) but it is also likely to be dangerous to the rehabilitation of invalids who are not naturally strong minded and who may therefore come to rely on being cared for and cossetted to their own – and their family's or attendant's – ultimate cost.

For people whose physical disability is due to an illness, like a stroke or an accident, rehabilitation in as many spheres of life as possible should be the aim. For others, it is at least as important to adapt positively as far as they can to their handicap. Even learning how to eat, dress or care for themselves, however slowly, is a help in regaining a sense of identity, independence, and, finally, self-respect.

Home is the background against which people relate to find themselves and their role in the community. For a disabled father or mother of a family, it is the place where they can continue to play their part in the family unit. Even for elderly people living alone, it is the place where they can be surrounded by their own possessions and the memories enshrined in these, despite the fact that the glass-fronted cabinet, or the brass-railed bed have been transferred from the home where they once lived to the bungalow or flat where they are now.

But if grown-up sons or daughters, physically disabled but still capable of looking after themselves independently, and maybe even to hold down an outside job, feel that they have the ability and the opportunity to leave the parental roof and set up their own establishments, this should not be anxiously opposed. Life is already difficult enough for young people who are physically disabled, and thereby excluded from living like their contemporaries and maybe having families of their own. In any case, their move to independence away from their parents may only be an intelligent anticipation of the state of affairs when ageing parents may later on be no longer available or able to look after their disabled child.

The most important feature is to make the home safe and easy to run.

A purpose-built home sounds ideal for a physically handicapped person: preferably a place where stairs, windows, doorways and rooms are suited to his requirements. A settlement of specially-designed bungalows clustered round a day-care centre is a solution which is now being tried out especially in situations where a physically-disabled person is married to an able-bodied partner. He or she can then go out to work each day, knowing that the disabled husband or wife can either attend the centre or be visited on demand by a member of the centre's staff.

It sounds ideal and it can work well: a disabled housewife, for instance, may sit in a wheelchair in her own, specially-adapted home with no stairs, perhaps doing the housework at her own leisurely pace or preparing the evening meal, with an occasional neighbour popping in to make sure she's all right.

But the reality does not always work out this way. Many experienced social workers hesitate to recommend a move to someone elderly or newly disabled, because this may mean the loss of faithful local friends and neighbours, as well as the shops, clinics, libraries, etc. where he is known. Moving house can be an ordeal at any time in one's life, but if it also entails giving up a whole satisfactory way of living, the reasons for it must be very strong to prevail.

Not that running even a much-loved home should ever be allowed to become an intolerable burden. Everyone's health and energy fluctuates occasionally, even more so in the case of a sufferer from certain illnesses or physical disabilities. Housework which has to be performed against a background of actual pain should be cut to the barest minimum. It is far better – and more efficient too – to leave the washing or the cleaning for a day or so when necessary. Even getting up can be deferred for a few hours, or maybe a whole day, if one isn't feeling quite up to it.

An emergency routine for such below-standard days is a great standby: a telephone near the bed to call a relative or a friend to help, to summon the doctor, the district nurse, or merely ask the local shopkeeper to send in food.

Emergency calls

It's only common sense to plan for the worst – while hoping it will never happen.

If you're suddenly taken ill, who's going to know about it – especially if you're living on your own?

Make sure the tradesmen who call know you and your circumstances. The paperboy, the milkman, or the porter of a block of flats can summon help if you've asked them to look out for you when they come round, especially if you make a point of chatting to them whenever you see them, and reinforce this with a packet of cigarettes or small tip at Christmas or at holiday time. You're not making a fuss, nor are you being a nuisance, and you would cause far more trouble to everyone concerned if they don't find you in good time to do what is necessary.

Better still, if you can make some personal arrangement with a neighbour to call in at the same time each morning, say, when she's on her way out to the shops. Or get into the habit of telephoning a friend or a relative each day at the same time. You needn't make a lengthy conversation of this, it's just a way of letting her know positively that you're all right. Then, if you don't phone, she'll know that something is wrong and can try to contact you or to get help.

No telephone? No friends? No neighbours? As a long-term measure, try to get to know someone who lives near you, even if it's only to smile and say good morning out of the window.

But don't necessarily wait until the new contact has ripened into a real friendship: take the first step by chatting to them, and explaining your situation. Most people are quite happy to take on a responsibility towards a neighbour in this way.

Get yourself a sign to put in the window and have it ready somewhere, just in case. Write HELP on it in large letters, using paint, or coal, or a lipstick, and make sure it's large and legible. A large envelope is good, and if you can stick it in the middle of the window-pane with Scotch tape, so much the better. It would alert a neighbour, especially if they realize you're on your own. You might even agree a light signal with them, for use at night. Some elderly people wear whistles, to blow in case of emergency. And in some areas local Rotary Clubs run special emergency call schemes for house-bound people.

Outside the house, have you made sure that even a passing stranger could help you if he were the first to find you? Carry your name and address in your wallet or handbag. Have a note of your doctor or the hospital where you are or have been treated. Stick it where it can be seen in your home too: in the drawer of a writing-table, or behind an ornament on the mantelpiece.

One simple precaution in case of accident or sudden illness is to enable other people to get into your home. A key given to a friend or neighbour or tucked unobtrusively inside a flowerpot or under a doormat is a safety measure so that an outsider can let himself into the house when necessary, or if no answer has been received to a phone call or knock on the door. For deaf people who may not hear the bell even if someone is ringing it, an electric or battery system of lights can be connected up. Often, local welfare departments will install these. The Royal National Institute for the Deaf has a list of useful appliances.

For the less mobile, a key on a long string can be lowered out of the window in answer to a caller, provided you've heard him, and are able to get to the window but not to the front door.

Many superstitious people seem to think that planning for an emergency is tantamount to meeting trouble half-way. If you're inclined that way, just ask yourself: 'What would happen if I fainted or broke a leg or simply found one morning that I couldn't get up?' You won't want to wait then, or don't you mind?

Some local authorities are already providing free telephones for elderly housebound people. It may be worth checking whether yours has decided to follow suit as it is intended councils should under the Chronically Sick and Disabled Persons Act.

Telephones for the disabled

For many house-bound people, the telephone is the vital link with the outside world. The GPO is aware of this special need of a small sub-section of telephone users and suggests that subscribers who cannot use their telephones because of a physical disability should get a friend to contact the local telephone manager by asking the operator to put them through. It's a service call and shouldn't even cost anything. He may be able to help them in all sorts of unexpected ways.

Certain standard aids for the deaf are readily available, including an amplifying handset which looks like an ordinary receiver and boosts incoming speech. The volume can be controlled by a thumb wheel near the ear piece, and the whole appliance can equally well be used without the amplification. The connecting fee is £1 10s. 0d., the additional charge 10s. 0d. per quarter. Special loud-ringing bells over a wide range of sound to suit varying forms of deafness can be fitted into a telephone at a charge of 3s. 0d. per quarter, or a combination of light signals (flashing or continuous) may be even more suitable. The quarterly charge is 5s. 0d.

For blind or partially sighted telephone users, a marked dial with raised marks on the outside indicating numbers 4 and 7 could be useful. All modern telephones are now fitted with a larger dial number ring to help elderly people with failing eyesight. These rings can also be fitted onto an existing telephone.

For people suffering from loss of voice, a faint speech amplifier would add £1 to the quarterly telephone bill and cost £2 to connect in the first place.

Finally, for anyone with disabled hands or unable to hold the telephone to their ear, there are a number of solutions—especially useful in the future as more and more calls will have to be made by dialling which might present them with insurmountable difficulties. A *Sender No. 1* consists of a separate small box from which the operator can be contacted direct by means of a press-button. This is supplied free to the physically disabled. Commercial telephone amplifiers which need not be held to the ear because they amplify incoming and outgoing speech can be bought at prices between £4 and £19 19s. 0d. The Research Institute for Consumer Affairs has published *Telephones and The Private Subscriber*, by Michael Dunne which provides details of where these can be bought.

Adapting one's home

A purpose-built home may sound ideal for the physically disabled. Many of the practical features to be described in this book should be found already built in which certainly cuts out a lot of planning and worry.

But there's also much to be said for remaining in a home you know, where you've been happy so far. Quite a lot can be done to make an existing, apparently awkward, home suitable to your special needs.

This is a matter for an expert: not just a builder or an architect, nor the local authority who may be paying for the alteration, nor even the disabled person for whom it is intended.

Two books which may be useful are:

An Introduction to Domestic Design for the Disabled by Felix Walter, FRIBA, FRSA, 12s. 6d. from the Disabled Living Foundation, and *Designing for the Disabled*, by Selwyn Goldsmith, published by the RIBA at £3 10s.

Although these books are mainly aimed at local authorities and people concerned with building new homes for the disabled, they contain many suggestions about the siting of storage units, sinks, light switches and socket outlets, special adaptations for the chairbound as regards doorways, ramps, bathrooms and WCs and so on, which would be equally useful for those who want to improve their own home.

Adequate housing is basic to happiness; for the housebound almost more than for other people. The most important points to watch out for are safety, convenience, warmth and, if possible, the opportunity to be independent about visiting the WC, having a bath, washing, cleaning the house and cooking.

Obviously, the specific arrangements of the home must depend on the nature of the occupant's handicap and whether he or she lives alone or has someone to help. People in wheelchairs must have space to move from room to room, including the bathroom, and to transfer into and out of it where necessary, either independently, or with help (human, a handrail, or an electric hoist). Doorways must be measured before the wheelchair is bought. Often, they need to be made wider.

Generally speaking, people in wheelchairs and those who have difficulty in walking, but manage with crutches, find life in a ground-floor room or flat more satisfactory than one higher up, even if there is a lift to take them there. A lift out of commission, however temporarily, would have an utterly paralysing effect, producing a feeling of being imprisoned. But in an existing household, the conversion of one downstairs room into a bed-sitting room would be a relatively simple alteration. Obviously, convenient washing and toilet facilities will also have to be provided.

Sometimes an elderly or arthritic person may have some difficulty in negotiating stairs, especially if they are relatively steep and necessitate a major hip movement. Grandiose schemes for electric lifts or hoists may seem out of the question (write to Hammond & Champness Ltd., 159 St John's Street, London, EC1 for a brochure if they're not and prepare to spend £700–£1,000), but a gadget like a moveable half-stair (see Fig. 1) may reduce the dreaded distance to something the invalid can cope with. This ingenious contraption can be moved up or down each stair by means of a stick. It can be ordered through the British Red Cross Society's local branch (find their address in your local telephone directory), who will normally send a representative to look over the premises and the invalid before equipping him with the desired stair-climbing aid. They stress that it is *not* recommended in every case but will provide it where it's likely to be useful, at a charge of £1 3s. 0d.

Another major domestic difficulty suffered by many disabled people is that they cannot open or shut windows when they are on their own. Horizontal sliding windows, though expensive, are suggested as a solution which suits in quite a few cases, and narrow vertically-pivoted windows are also often used success-

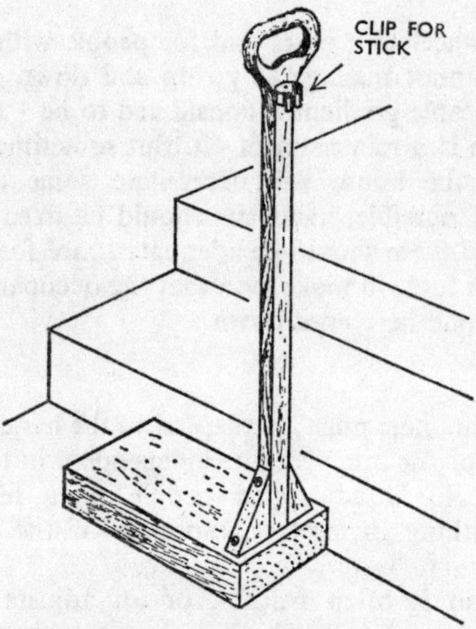

Fig. 1 Moveable half-stair. Instructions for use: 1. Put the half-step on the floor against the bottom step of the stairs. 2. Put both feet on it. The tread of the bottom step is then only 3½" higher than this level. 3. Step on the bottom step with one foot and then bring the second foot up. 4. Lift the portable half-step on to the bottom step beside you. 5. Repeat the action all the way up the steps or stairs. (From *Your Home and Your Rheumatism,* published by The Arthritis and Rheumatism Council.)

fully, provided that they do not protrude too much into the room.

Round door-knobs are difficult to manipulate for many physically handicapped people. They could be replaced by the lever kind.

Handrails

Probably the simplest alteration to make home life easier and safer is the installation of handrails on stairways, passages, in WCs, and bathrooms. Nylon-coated steel tubes are comfortable and easy to grip and they are less likely to split than the wooden kind.

Ramps

These are for wheelchair users and for people with walking difficulties who cannot manage to go up and down stairs.

The most suitable gradient is considered to be 1 in 12, and the preferred width is a minimum of 4ft. But sometimes the existing dimensions of the house will necessitate some alterations to these figures. If possible, handrails should be fixed on each side of the ramp and there should be adequate space for a wheelchair to run out at its foot, to make sure that the occupant will not get bumped each time he comes down.

Bathrooms

The arrangements here must be adapted to the handicapped user, especially if he or she intends to be independent in the bathroom.

Some physically handicapped people have relatively little difficulty in bathing themselves, especially if the equipment is right.

A low-set tub is often helpful, or an adjustable bath rail which can be screwed to the bath makes it easier to get in and out, especially if there is another grip on the corresponding side. A rubber mat in the tub (14s. 6d. Rubbermaid from Selfridges or J. & A. Carters – for address see Appendix) reduces the risk of slipping, or an adjustable bath seat, made from wood, steel tubing or aluminium, means that sitting down and getting up will not necessitate a vast change of levels. Most such seats are provided with rubber protectors to avoid marking the bath (Army & Navy Stores). An ordinary bathroom stool, cork-seated, is a useful device for getting in and out of the tub, too, though a more severely disabled person may need a special ceiling hoist for this, with which the local authority may be able to help.

If a shower is available, this is often a suitable washing convenience for an elderly person who finds getting in and out of the bath too difficult. A shower chair, rather like a toilet seat on legs (£4 15s. 0d. from J. & A. Carters) or a more solid armchair on wheels (mobile shower chair, £16 10s. 0d. from J. & A. Carters) means that they can sit while they wash.

Turning a tap can be difficult for some physically disabled people. A long-handled lever tap fitment is much easier to handle than a conventional four-pronged top and can be added to any tap made since 1944 (Lever Tap conversion unit from Leva Tap Company, £1 5s. 0d. to £1 10s. 0d.). A simpler but fairly effective tap turner for an old-fashioned tap can even be home-made from a piece of wood with four screws in the head to fit over the prongs of the tap top (Fig. 2).

For the bathroom floor, cork is recommended. This useful material is warm to the feet and isn't slippery even when wet. An emergency door lock, which can be opened from the outside in case of accident, can be useful. A simple nylon bolt (3s. 0d. from the Army & Navy Stores) or the Stirling Suite Bathroom door set (35s. 0d. from Hobbs of Whitefriars Street, London, EC4) means that a child or disabled adult can be rescued even if they can't re-open the locked door for themselves.

WCs

Not surprisingly, for most elderly and physically handicapped people the ability to use the WC independently is a jealously-guarded dignity. It is, after all, a child's first intimation of independence from mother so that abdicating from it for anything except the most transitory of periods seems a very final gesture. Everything possible should therefore be done to allow even a severely disabled person to cope, although this may take an unusually long time.

For the chairbound, a visit to the WC can mean a complicated transfer operation. The chair need not necessarily be brought further than the door, as many people retain the ability to slide out of it – leaving the door open and helping themselves with handrails until they reach their objective. If necessary, and possible, the wheelchair can also be brought right into the WC so that the user can slide out of it and onto the WC, using it astride, facing the rear wall. If the wheelchair has a collapsible or sliding armrest this operation can also be undertaken sideways.

The lavatory seat should preferably be about the same height as that of the wheelchair. Many disabled people, arthritics, for instance, also find a raised lavatory more comfortable to use. Special lavatory seats can be bought (i.e. from the British Red Cross Society at £1 18s. 0d.) to put on an existing lavatory to get the necessary height to suit those who are stiff and find bending and stooping painful or even impossible. For them, a

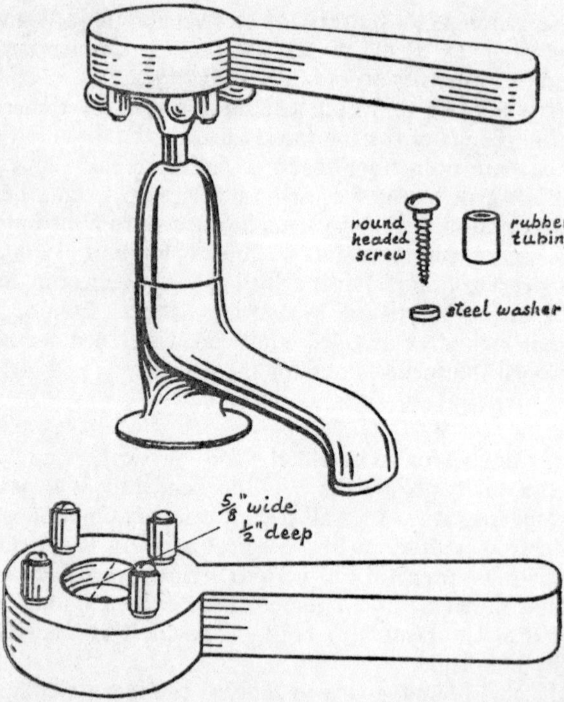

Fig. 2 Tap Turner. Materials required: a piece of smooth wood; four 1½" steel washers; a piece of rubber (gas) tubing about 4" long. From a piece of hard wood (beech, ash or mahogany) 1" thick, cut out the shape of the tap turner as per diagram, in one piece, with a fretsaw. (Overall length about 6¾", diameter of circular head 2½".) With a ⅝" gimlet, hollow out the centre of the circular head to a depth of about ½" to fit over the domed part on a tap handle, and to allow the tap turner to rotate more freely. Next, mark off the positions for the four screws on the circular head, making sure that these are spaced correctly to correspond with the spaces between the prongs on the handle of a tap. Make the four holes for the screws first with a small ⅛" drill to a depth of about ⅝". These holes must be drilled first of all, before the screws are inserted, or the wood will spilt. Slip the steel washers on to the round-headed screws and push up to under the heads. Cut the rubber (gas) tubing in lengths of about ¾", and slip them over the screws, pushing them up to meet the washers. Put a smear of soap on the screw-threads, to help them to go in more easily. Then screw them gently into the holes prepared for them to a depth of approximately ⅝". (From *Home-made Aids for the Disabled,* published by the British Red Cross Society.)

special grip rail (like one by Goslett, at £12 18s. 0d.) surrounding the WC makes getting up no more difficult than getting out of an armchair.

Of course, adapting a WC can be a time-consuming operation. While waiting to have an existing lavatory adapted or a new one installed, a commode can be hired or borrowed from the local authority or branch of the British Red Cross.

A pricey but ingenious WC-cum-bidet incorporating a foot button which activates warm-water cleansing followed by a warm air drier (£258 from Clos-O-Mat Ltd, 2 Brooklands Road, Sale, Cheshire M33 355) has been installed in some private homes for the limbless and other physically handicapped people.

Kitchens

Everything that applies to kitchen planning for normal housewives also applies to the physically disabled, only more so. Some splendid ideal solutions have been worked out – but how few housewives are lucky enough to own an ideal kitchen? Furthermore their requirements will vary, not only according to their physical disability but according to the amount of cooking and housekeeping they are likely to do and whether they enjoy this as a personal hobby and fulfilment or find it just another chore to get through.

A chairbound woman may well be able to work in her kitchen, provided there is enough space for her to move about in and if the working-top is set low and the sink not only low but shallow. Obviously, for one with reduced reach the storage cupboards should be placed low too and kitchen tools accessible in a drawer or suspended on a peg-board. A split-level oven which can be set at a convenient height is useful, and so is a built-in refrigerator which can more easily be used and cleaned than one standing on the floor. Electric boiling rings with safety rims can be set into table tops, and a safety rim like the Gayleigh cooker safeguard (£4 10s. 0d to £5 10s. 0d. from Gas and Electricity Boards showrooms) is child-proof as well as invalid-proof when fixed on either side of the cooking surface to make sure that saucepans are not pulled off or slid off inadvertently.

A great deal of special kitchen equipment is available for the disabled. There are, for instance, ingenious, specially-designed knives, forks and spoons with thickened or curved handles which can be obtained for between 5s. 0d. and 7s. 0d. from the British Red Cross, whose illustrated catalogue *Aids for the Disabled* costs 4s. 0d., plus postage. This also contains descriptions of stands from which beakers can be tilted for drinking, and other drinking aids, a plate surround to make sure that food does not get pushed off the plate, and a teapot stand and plate holder to help people with uncertain muscular co-ordination or a deficiency in the hand. One tip worth noting is that the bottoms of the ordinary table dishes and plates can be covered with foam rubber to prevent slipping about on trays or tables. A layer of foam rubber on flat surfaces like these also acts as a stabilizer. For 49s. 6d., Melaware Ltd. make a specially designed set of eating utensils in practical, break-resistant Melamine consisting of two tilted plates with rims, an easy-to-grasp beaker and thick-handled, short-headed knives, forks and spoons. These are useful for arthritics and spastics and are available from Boots.

Some adaptations of everyday kitchen or eating utensils are well within the scope of the average family handyman. For anyone who finds normal-weight cutlery too heavy to use, plastic or perspex spoons can be given an easy-grip loop of garter elastic (see Fig. 3 for instructions). Enlarged handgrips for cutlery can be made from foam rubber tubing, Rubazote, which you should be able to get from the Welfare Department of your local council. Another way to enlarge the handles of knives is to substitute for them Wangee cane (sold by Jacobs Young and Westbury, Bridge Road, Haywards Heath, Sussex). Each length makes three handles. Two ingenious home-made drinking aids on the principle of a bent drinking straw are also suggested in *Home-made Aids for the Disabled* for people who can't use a cup or bend their necks.

Another useful handbook and buying guide of kitchen equipment is *List of Kitchen Equipment*, published by the Disabled Living Foundation at 5s. 9d. It features everyday items from tin-openers and knives for the one-handed (Nelson knife, 11s. 6d. from Hugh Steeper Ltd, Roehampton Lane, London, SW15) to specially-stabilized mixing bowls made of rubber as well as an ingenious device to prevent milk from boiling over (Solidex

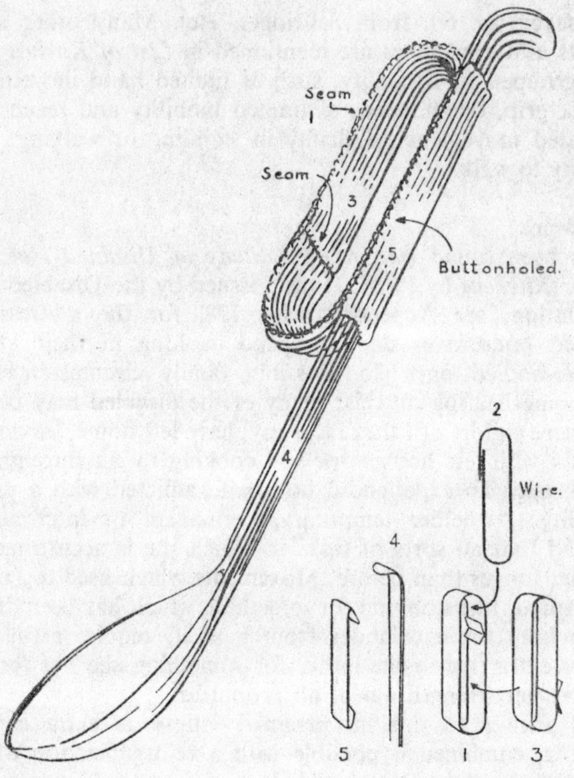

Fig. 3 Easy-grip spoon. You will require sufficient garter elastic to go twice round the patient's hand and allowing for turnings. Cut in half and join up separately (1 and 3). These will eventually be buttonholed together along the edges, one inside the other, to form the hand-loop. In addition, a small piece of the elastic about 2½–3″ long is required (5) to join to the hand-loop making the slot through which the handle of the spoon is passed. As will be seen in the diagram, the hand-loop is reinforced between the double thicknesses of elastic with a piece of steel wire (or a piece of an old clock spring can be used for this), bent round to the correct size (2). This is important as it prevents the elastic from sagging and keeps the loop open for the patient's hand to be slipped through easily. (From *Home-made Aids for the Disabled*, published by the British Red Cross Society.)

milk saver, 3s. 6d. from Selfridges, etc). Many other kitchen gadgets and appliances are mentioned in *List of Kitchen Equipment* grouped by disability, such as limited hand movement or a weak grip, one-handed, of limited mobility and reach, uncoordinated movements, difficulty in standing or walking, or the inability to walk.

Housework

It has been found (see *A Pilot Study of Disabled Housewives in their Kitchens* by P. M. Howie, issued by the Disabled Living Foundation, see Appendix, page 128, for the address) that disabled housewives do not spend as long in their kitchens as able-bodied ones do. Possibly family circumstances may have some bearing on this: many of the disabled may be of an age where children (if they have any) have left home, leaving their mothers with less housework and cooking to get through.

Still, even an experienced housewife afflicted with a physical disability – whether temporary, permanent or intermittent – will find that all sorts of tasks to which she is accustomed will take her longer than before. Movements which used to be taken for granted, like stooping for something which has been dropped or reaching for a colander from a shelf, require great effort, and an extra trip to the larder for something she has forgotten may tax her strength out of all proportion.

The answer to this unwarranted fatigue is extra care and planning, combined if possible with a re-organization of tasks previously considered essential. Is it, for example, necessary to peel the potatoes? And must all the stores really be kept in a cupboard which may be out of reach? Assembling on a trolley all the materials for an operation like cooking a meal may eliminate a number of wearying trips to the larder, fridge and store cupboard.

Cooking a hot meal for one's husband or family is part of a housewife's home-making function. It may make her feel happy to be still of active use to her nearest and dearest, but this does not mean that it must be a full-scale effort, including numerous dishes and followed by a cooked dessert. Family meals do not only consist of food but also provide an opportunity to sit down together and mull over the events of the day. Disabled housewives should therefore not hesitate to make full use of all the ready-prepared and easy-to-make foods they can get: ready-made soups in tins, sauces in tins or tubes, packaged soups and sauces, meat pre-cut or ready-minced for immediate cooking, sliced bread and cheese, frozen vegetables which require no preparation, yoghourts and ice-cream desserts and many others. A wall-mounted tea dispenser like the Caddymatic (6s. 11d. from Selfridges and other stores) is operated by a push button and obviates the need to open a tin and fiddle with a spoon each time tea is made.

Blind or partially-sighted housewives must learn to be particularly methodical in the kitchen. A leaflet *Hints for Blind Housewives* is available from the RNIB and suggests that practice in making tea with a measured amount of water in the kettle and in draining vegetables with a colander will streamline many cooking operations which might otherwise be hazardous. Special braille knobs can be fitted to cookers, refrigerators and timers, and heavy-weight pans are recommended for those who feel that a meal is not a meal unless some part of it is fried. Maybe a little information about the calorific content of fried foods would help too on this score: house-bound people should pay particular attention to their diet to make sure they don't get unnecessarily fat or constipated. (If you're not sure what foods make you put on weight, send a stamped, addressed envelope to *Woman*, Beauty Department, 185 High Holborn, London, WC1 for their slimming leaflet which categorizes food by calorie content.)

Avoiding fatigue

Often the simplest ideas are the ones which save most time and trouble, like fixing a wire basket underneath your letter-box to make sure you don't have to bend down to the door-mat every time the postman has been.

A simple tilting table of adjustable height (i.e. New Cantilever Table, £5 17s. 6d. from John Lewis and other stores) can be used by a chair-bound or even bed-bound patient for reading and writing. If mounted on castors it can be moved away when it is no longer wanted.

That sturdy shopping basket on wheels can be as useful in ferrying things from one room to the other as it is for bringing home one's purchases, whether you baulk at carrying heavy loads or any loads whatsoever. A special walking-aid trolley for housewives from the Army & Navy Stores (Victoria Street, London, SW1) costing 16 guineas is a bulk transporter for anyone with a weak grip or uncertain walk.

A long-handled dustpan and brush set (from Homecraft Supplies Ltd, 27 Trinity Road, London, SW17 or from Medor Ltd, 80 Copenhagen Street, Caledonian Road, London, N1) means that the floor can be swept without stooping. Brooms should be lightweight and can, if necessary, be fitted with an elbow crutch to give better control at long distance. A light-weight carpet sweeper may be easier and less tiring to use round the house than a full-scale vacuum cleaner, although it's no use pretending that it has quite the same effect on anything other than a few crumbs or cigarette ash on the carpet.

Nowadays few able-bodied housewives think of getting down on their knees for the cleaning, so why shouldn't the disabled profit from the back- and knee-saving items which are available: the self-wringing sponge mop for the floor and the self-wringing window cleaner?

If you haven't got a washing-machine, try to organize somebody to go to the launderette for you. If your ironing-board is too high to sit at, try to get one of those tall kitchen stools (about 30in high), preferably with a back-rest (from large stores, i.e. the John Lewis group, £6 to £7). This is also a fatigue-saver when you're cooking, as you can sit down to some of those tasks using the cooker or 3ft-high working surfaces, like stirring food or preparing vegetables.

Shopping

Be sensible about shopping: not just about the things you buy but the way you buy them.

Fortunately mail order is becoming better by the month and more and more people take advantage of it for buying clothes, household appliances, furniture and food. Bulk orders are fine and economical, provided you have storage space and someone to take in the parcels for you: John Dron (Mountview House, London, N6) have a catalogue full of useful and solid household goods for you to choose from; Nylons Unlimited (Gay Street,

Bath, Somerset) have branched out beyond stockings and panti-tights to undies and knitwear; and various mail-order specialists (like Kays of Worcester, for instance) will send you 100-page illustrated catalogues of department-store goods to pick for yourself or – at a useful discount to yourself – for family members and friends. You can pick up quite reasonable bargains from those unexciting and crowded small-ads. pages in newspapers too.

The telephone is a great help to the home-bound shopper. It's quite safe to order branded goods by telephone from even the grandest stores, although the abolition of retail price maintenance means that they're sometimes a bit more expensive than the ones you could have bought for yourself at Boots or Woolworths. Still, you'll be saving the price of a bus fare or petrol for the car which may help to close the gap.

Most large stores send catalogues to account customers, but one shop which specializes in a mail-order service for the disabled is the Army & Navy Stores, Victoria Street, London, SW1. Write to them for their shopping list which has been compiled in conjunction with the Disabled Living Foundation. Another service they provide is wheelchair transport for personal shoppers throughout their store.

For more information about shopping in person see p. 94 in Chapter 4, Getting round and about.

Bedrooms

It would be nice to plan a bedroom from scratch, especially for someone who may have to spend all or at least a large part of every day there. Such a bedroom may have to be his or her whole world, providing if at all possible a view through the window (if the bed is high or the window low enough) and a collection of anything the patient is likely to need near his bed: radio or television, bell, a typewriter or writing materials, books, knitting, etc.

A suitable bed is important, especially to a person who may not be able to sit up unaided. A special bed can give him at least a minimum of mobility and enable him to sit up or at an angle. An electrically-powered bed can turn him over, too. Obviously such beds have to be bought specially and can be chosen through *Equipment for the Disabled*, already mentioned on page 21. This contains a comprehensive section on special beds as well as hoists and other bedroom equipment.

Fortunately, not all the physically disabled are entirely supine. A special drawer under the bed is equally useful for the bed-bound and for the partially mobile who can keep their clothes in it and dress, sitting or lying on the bed, even if someone else may have to stoop and open it for them (see Fig. 4). At least, everything they need is there together.

Bed-making will be easier if fitted sheets are used. A chair-bound housewife can make the bed if there is a space round it: about 3ft clear is suggested. Beds on castors are easy to move about for cleaning, but one of the castors should have a simple brake attachment to make sure it does not slide about when its occupant is about to retire, possibly wearily, for a rest.

A telephone or alarm bell to connect with the outside is useful to have near the bed in case of emergency.

Ordinary alarm clocks may present difficulties for people who are deaf or hard of hearing. The Royal National Institute for the Deaf (105 Gower Street, London, WC1) have a flashing alarm clock (Callaflash, 57s. 6d.) but a really heavy sleeper may need their vibratory pillow (90s.) in addition. This is plugged into a Callaflash-type alarm clock and should shake him into waking up.

Heating

One man's ideal temperature is another man's idea of a stuffy fug, but the disabled are generally likely to require more heat than someone whose circulation is kept going by moving about and taking exercise. A temperature ranging from 65°–72° F should be aimed at, if at all possible, with special provision to keep the feet and lower limbs warm.

Unfortunately, heating is expensive. One small economy which can be practised is to make sure that heat is not lost through insufficient insulation in the house. Draughts can be eliminated with double glazing or heavy curtaining. People in wheelchairs often leave doors open, which means that the entire living-space should be heated to the desired temperature.

Obviously, no disabled person should ever be exposed to the risk of fire. Coal and gas fires must be properly screened. Electric

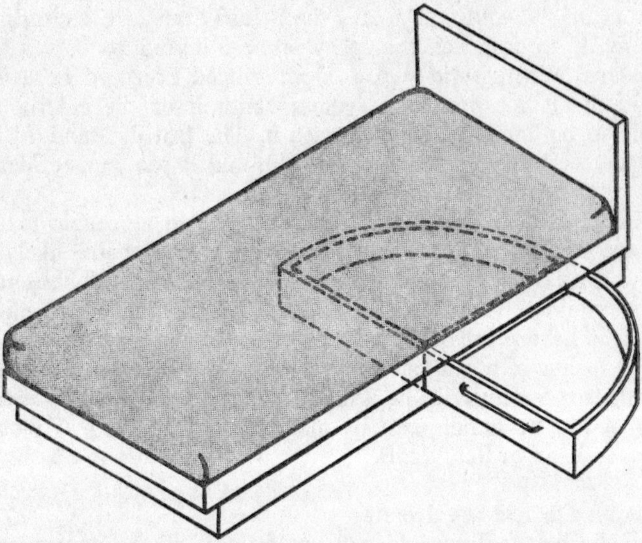

Fig. 4 Quadrant drawer beneath the bed. (From *An Introduction to Domestic Design for the Disabled,* by Felix Walter, FRIBA, published by the Disabled Living Foundation.)

night-storage heaters are useful and should not make too large a hole in the weekly budget. The heat they provide can be topped up by convector heaters or closed solid-fuel stoves when required. Oil heaters are sometimes in the news because they have caused accidents, but they are a relatively inexpensive source of heat and need not necessarily be ruled out provided they are used with due care. The Royal Society for the Prevention of Accidents suggest that all oil heaters should be firmly positioned or even fixed so that they can't topple over, that they should be made to stand on some fireproof surround of brick or stone or even merely a square tin lid and that the greatest care is taken in filling them without spilling inflammable paraffin. All oil heaters sold in the UK during the last eight years or so have been made to British

Standard 3300, and many carry the British Standard Institution's Kitemark to indicate that they've been tested to this safety standard. Where solid fuel is used, a fixed fireguard is always recommended, especially if young children or the elderly are likely to be left on their own with it. The British Standard for this nursery-type fireguard is BS3140, and it too can be identified by the Kitemark.

Heating the bathroom and WC may be an agreeable luxury for the able-bodied, but for disabled people who are likely to spend a great deal more time in these places it is really essential to maintain a reasonable temperature level. Wall- or ceiling-mounted heaters are quick to warm the room and can be switched on by means of a pull-cord. If the usual plastic knob at the end of this is too slender to be grasped by anyone with an uncertain grip, a thicker handle can be made with a padding of plastic foam over an ordinary cork.

Walking aids and wheelchairs

Even the best walking aid will not provide all the convenience and mobility of having one's own two legs. This is the reason why hospital consultants often hesitate to prescribe wheelchairs (which are available under the NHS) to seemingly quite disabled patients whom they are encouraging to learn to walk independently again.

Such training can be initiated in hospital or by a physiotherapist and amounts to using muscles hitherto neglected. Energy and perseverance with exercises which may be boring or even painful are essential. Often, quite remarkable success is achieved, even by patients recovering from a stroke or paralysis following an accident. If, therefore, the specialist has definitely refused to prescribe a walking aid or wheelchair, he is not necessarily being hardhearted or sadistic. He may simply be confident that real progress towards some physical independence is possible.

Sometimes elderly people living at home may not have brought their walking difficulties to the doctor's notice because the deterioration has been so gradual that they have not thought of calling him in, or they have not been sufficiently articulate in describing their problems when they were being seen by him.

If necessary, their walking problem should be brought to the doctor's notice by some relative or attendant. Probably quite a lot can be done to help.

Walking aids may be anything from a simple cane to a complicated walking platform on wheels. They include crutches to be used from elbow or shoulder, quadruped walking aids to be used like supporting sticks or trolleys which can be pushed by the patient and are, in fact, medical equipment to be obtained on medical advice.

Wheelchairs, too, vary widely from the light, home 'glide-about' manoeuvrable chair to a wide range of vehicles with various kinds of head-rests, arm-rests, leg-rests, a gap in the seat to accommodate a urinal, differently-positioned wheels, as well as special wheelchairs for disabilities like leg amputations. Electrically-powered wheelchairs (i.e. Bec or Powerdrive) provide mobility for quite severely disabled people at home and even in their gardens and beyond, but they cannot go up and down kerbs, which limits their outdoor use, even in good weather.

The choice is bewildering, especially as it often has to be made by a person other than the eventual user. The main guiding lines should be laid down by expert medical opinion of the patient's disability. The dimensions of his home and the doors he will have to negotiate are obviously also important factors. Second wheelchairs which may have to fold up to go into the boot of a certain make of car may also be necessary. The information service of the Disabled Living Foundation can advise on these. Carters sell a range of folding wheelchairs made by Everest & Jenning for anyone who is determined to shop independently, though it is again emphasized that the D.L.F. will advise on these too.

Spinal patients at Stoke Mandeville Hospital are mostly provided with one of the wheelchairs from the Zimmer range, Junior Standard, or with a semi-reclining back. There are also special 'growing chairs' for children made on the same principle as bicycles where the frames can be lengthened.

For any elderly person who resists the idea of using a wheelchair because he or she sees it as the ultimate sign of debility, it may be worth pointing out that the Department of Health and Social Security (who themselves issue over 80,000 wheelchairs under the NHS) estimate that more than one person in every 1,000 uses a wheelchair at some time in his life.

By far the greatest proportion of wheelchair users (over a quarter) suffer from some form of arthritis; the next largest group are people with organic muscular diseases like multiple sclerosis, etc. Disability does not necessarily spell age.

Eighty per cent of the Department-issued wheelchairs belong to the standard self-propelling type, folding wheelchairs, 15 per cent are folding outdoor chairs and 5 per cent are rigid-framed indoor chairs. But for some people electrically-powered indoor chairs mean a second chance to do a job or to run their own homes. Over 600 such chairs were provided by the Department in 1967 and others can, of course, be bought direct from suppliers of medical equipment.

Artificial limbs (Prostheses)

Someone you know may well be one of the 83,000 amputees, even if only his nearest and dearest realize it. About 73,000 (this includes the congenitally limbless, i.e. those who were born without one or several complete limbs) attend one of the twenty-eight regional Limb and Appliance Centres in the UK. Nine people need an artificial leg for every one requiring an artificial arm. And about 10,000 amputees have lost a finger or toe which probably doesn't need replacement for ordinary purposes, anyway.

The majority of lower limb amputees are elderly, and indeed some 63 per cent of all those who are referred to the limb-fitting service every year are over the age of 60. A high proportion have lost their legs through disease, notably diabetic and arterio-sclerotic gangrene; about 15 per cent have had an accident at work or on the roads; and a relatively modest 4.6 per cent suffer from congenital malformation.

Prescribing and fitting an artificial limb is always a matter for professionals: doctors, surgeons, limb-fitters, contractors (who manufacture the limb) and physiotherapists will follow each other in an established progression from the moment an artificial leg or arm has been decided upon – and sometimes, in the case of a planned amputation, even before that.

In the UK the whole operation has become more or less comprehensively standardized in all parts of the country under the NHS, although it is of course also possible to have a limb made privately at your own expense.

Under the NHS there are thirteen basic legs to choose from, depending on the site of the amputation, with approximately one hundred variations involving leg control, suspension and feet; and there are about twenty basic arms made in three versions, each with a range of functional appliances according to the purpose for which they are to be used. With different end-pieces clipped into the wrist-socket, wearers can continue to do their ordinary work whether this includes holding a blow-lamp or wielding a hammer, driving a car or using a spade. Housewives can be equipped to hold a potato, to knit, or to use a sewing-machine. Probably the most versatile of all the grabbing devices is the basic split hook, spring-loaded to open and shut. Dr Selig at the Roehampton Limb Fitting Centre says that he can probably produce a device for any but the most esoteric movements an armless man or woman may wish to execute. Most right-handed people who lose their right arm soon learn to make do with their left. But experienced limb-fitters suggest that in certain cases, say that of a carpenter wielding a saw, this is best done by the hand – even the 'wrong' hand – so as to expose only the artificial limb to the risk of further injury. An efficient saw-holding appliance can be fitted, if necessary.

Great care is taken to ensure that artificial limbs fit their wearers anatomically. For this reason detailed measurements or plaster casts are taken and the wearer is later trained at a walking- or arm-training clinic to make sure that he or she can use the prostheses safely and efficiently. But this is not the only point to consider. Success in wearing an artificial limb also depends greatly on the wearer himself: his general state of health, his age, aptitude and how strongly he feels about re-integrating into everyday life and activities. A duplicate limb is always supplied, as a spare.

Like any other appliance, artificial limbs need care and attention if they are to give reasonable service. If they break or get damaged they should be immediately returned to the limb-fitting centre for an overhaul and should not be put aside, as happens all too often, until the spare replacement limb is also worn out, leaving the unfortunate wearer without either.

Another point worth remembering is that a prosthesis will need regular overhauls and re-fits, no matter how meticulously it was fitted originally. It may be showing signs of wear and tear from regular daily use. It is equally likely that the fit is not what it was, maybe because the stump for which it was made has changed physically or because its wearer has grown fatter or thinner or his needs have changed. Children will need new limbs as they grow too big or too muscular for the old ones.

The patient's first walking exercises are usually held when he has been fitted with simple pylons. But the eventual artificial leg which is made for him individually can be a fairly sophisticated structure, capable of flexing and bending, and can certainly pass for the real thing, especially inside a trouser leg.

The problems of children without arms or with defective arms are particularly urgent. Carbon-dioxide-powered limbs are proving successful for such cases. Much has been written about myo-electric hands, but they are only suitable for people with below-elbow amputations and are generally found to be of less functional value than conventional shoulder-operated arms. Obviously, therefore, they are of no use to armless children.

It is sometimes said that wearers of artificial limbs are relatively lucky compared to so many other physically disabled people because they can continue to lead normal lives and live in their own homes without any major problems of reconstruction (though firm wall-grips in bathrooms and WCs are recommended). On the other hand, this very unobtrusiveness of the average artificial limb complicates life for its wearer. No one may think of offering him a seat in a swaying bus or make any allowance for him at work or at home. Many active amputees may prefer this state of affairs to being cosseted and fussed over, but sometimes the comparison is not only unfair but frustrating.

Of course, the wearing of an artificial limb is less complicated for a healthy patient who can be fitted with a moveable arm or leg on a shoulder or pelvic harness. He then activates it himself by moving an existing muscle.

But any man-made limb – no matter by whom it is worn – has certain limitations. It cannot transmit sensations of heat or cold, hardness or softness and so on. This is a drawback which particularly affects young children who learn about the world by touch (as well as in other ways). Parents of armless children sometimes solve this difficulty by encouraging them to use their feet instead.

Feet can become very versatile with training. One way to develop them is to leave the feet and toes bare as much as possible to enable them to move freely, and to supply the child with cut-out shoes and mitten-type socks so that using his feet need not be preceded by a major undressing operation. Some children are known to be able to feed themselves, write, paint, type, handle money and even embroider with their feet. Obviously they can retain these valuable skills in adult life.

During 1969 an artificial arm on a shoulder harness which conveys texture by means of sound was developed for eleven armless children in Edinburgh by a Medical Research Council team. This may eventually become available for special cases.

Possum

No, this isn't a quaint Australian animal! Possum stands for 'Patient-Operated Selector Mechanisms': an electronic form of control mechanism which enables severely disabled people to carry out a whole battery of activities with their mouths or with a minimal touch of hand or foot: to summon help, unlock a door at a distance, adjust a heater or a television set, and so on.

At present about 160–170 patients in the UK are considered so disabled that they qualify for a free issue of Possum from the Ministry of Health and Social Security, provided that their GP's recommendation for it is confirmed by a regional board and a local assessment board. Since no applications for Possums have come from some parts of the country, there is now at least a suspicion that some patients who would qualify for a free issue either do not know about it or have not been advised by their medical or welfare authorities to apply for it.

The main advantage of this elaborate device is that it makes even a bedbound paraplegic to some degree independent, especially if his machine has a telephone control with which he can contact his doctor, if necessary. Other useful features which can be included in Possum are a door-unlocking device and an inter-comm. with the front door, as well as control of a

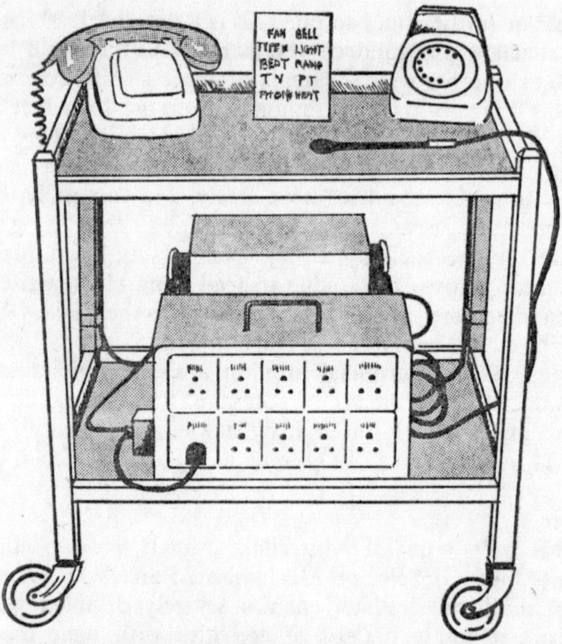

Fig. 5 POSSUM. Mobile equipment giving control over bell, light, radio, page-turner or micro-film projector, heat, telephone, television, bed tilt, (From the *Introductory Description* of Patient Operated Selector Mechanism Controls, distributed by POSM Research Project.)

bell, light, radio, page-turner or micro-film projector and heater (in the room or on an electric blanket).

Each machine is tailored to the individual invalid who will be using it and to the particular circumstances of his home. For further details, contact the makers: POSM Project Research, (63 Mandeville Road, Aylesbury, Bucks) who also manufacture the electronic typewriter which has enabled severely disabled people to resume earning their living as journalists, lawyers, computer specialists, etc. This, too, is available free, through the Department of Labour and Productivity to anyone who will use it professionally and can earn over £5 per week on it.

Bedbound

A bedbound patient should be receiving medical attention as well

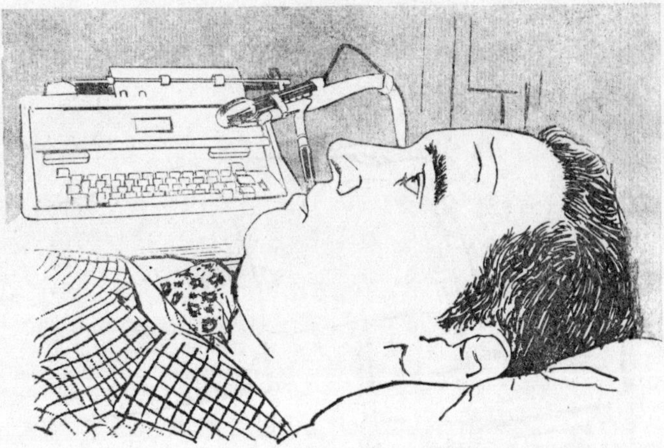

Fig. 6 POSSUM. Plastic pneumatic control tube being used to operate, by suction or pressure, a type-writer. (From the *Introductory Description* of Patient Operated Selector Mechanism Controls, distributed by POSM Research Project.)

as any practical advice he may need from the district nurse or welfare visitor. There are, however, some simple things which can be done to make a bedbound patient more comfortable and independent.

A home-made bed-tidy (see Fig. 7) consists of a strip of firm textile material, long enough to cover the width of a bed like a bedspread and hang down at least 18in on either side. Pockets are sewn on to it in various accessible positions, so that useful articles like a comb, face-cloth in a pocket lined with jaconet, book, writing materials, knitting, etc. can be kept within reach. The centre pocket should contain some stiff surface like a firm piece of cardboard, plywood or plastic so as to form a useful writing-board. A small strip of material sewn on at the appropriate place keeps the electric bell within easy reach.

Another useful item which is freely available in hospital but sometimes difficult to find for use at home is a bed-cradle (£2 8s. 0d. from Carters), to protect the patient from the pressure of blankets. Or an adjustable foot-rest (£4 15s. 0d.) can be

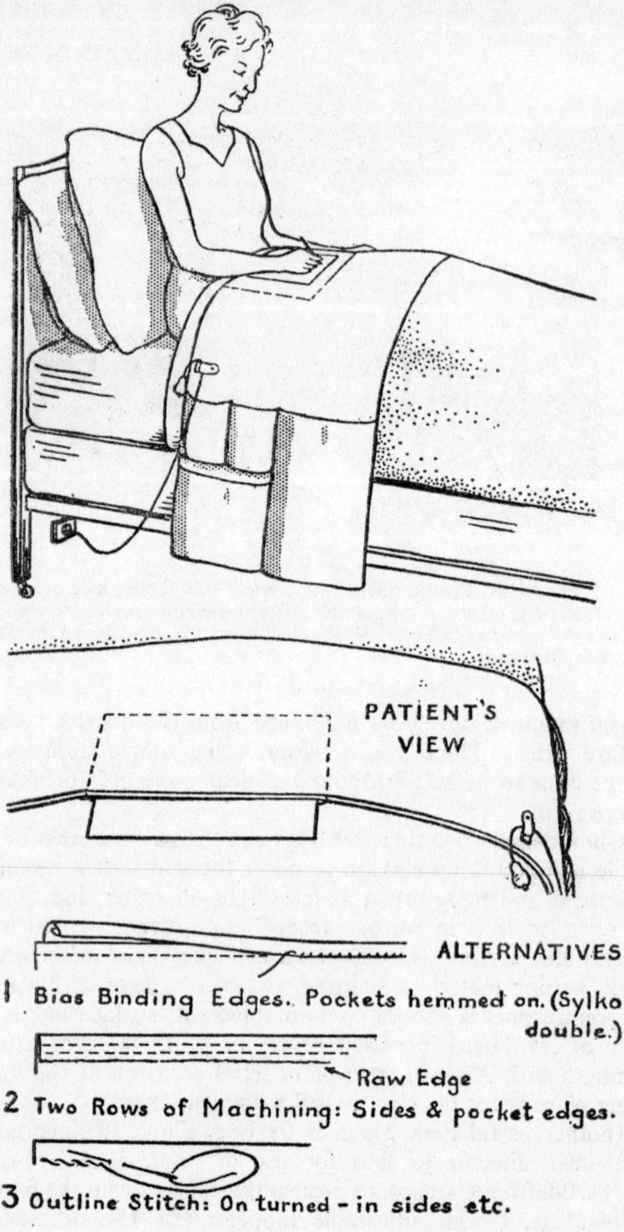

PATIENT'S VIEW
ALTERNATIVES
1 Bias Binding Edges. Pockets hemmed on. (Sylko double.)
Raw Edge
2 Two Rows of Machining: Sides & pocket edges.
3 Outline Stitch: On turned - in sides etc.

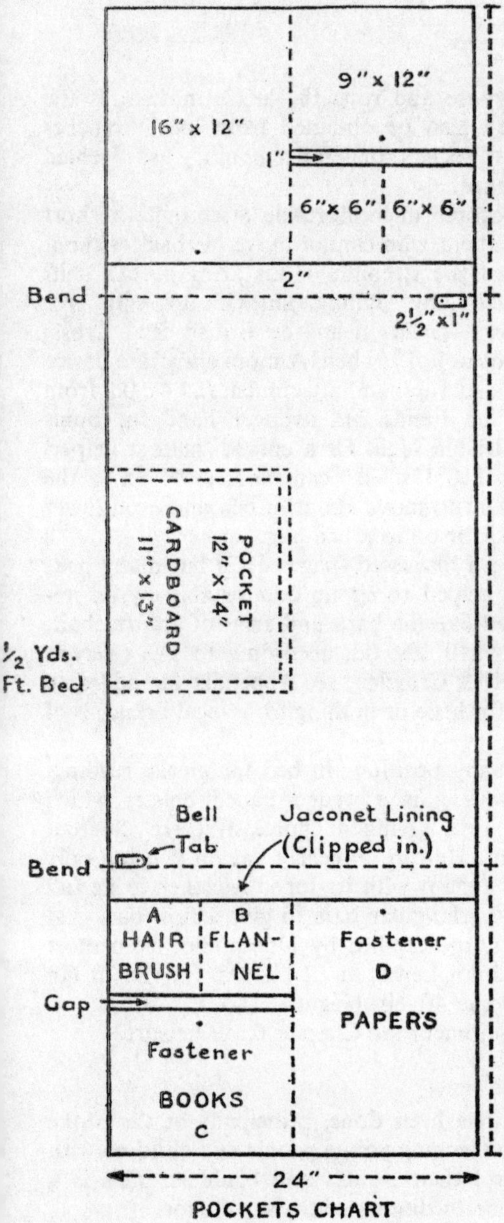

Fig. 7 Bed-tidy. The Tidy is devised to keep everything within reach for a bedridden patient. It is made out of a length of material sufficient to go across the bed and hang down at least 18" on either side. The pockets are made in different sizes to hold various articles: for example, a large pocket on the Tidy, hanging over the right of the bed, is for newspapers; two small pockets take a handkerchief and a comb; others can be made as required to hold a pen, pencil and a face cloth (the pocket for the latter should be lined with jaconet). In the centre of the Tidy is a pocket into which a firm piece of cardboard is slipped to act as a writing-board, and, as can be seen from the diagram, a small strip of material, sewn on at the appropriate place and fastening with a press-stud, keeps the electric bell in a handy place within easy reach for the patient. (Add ⅛" to the sizes given to allow for turnings.) (From *Home-made Aids for the Disabled,* published by the British Red Cross Society.)

used for the same purpose and rests the ankle muscles at the same time. Cradles can also be obtained from local branches of the British Red Cross Society, or – for temporary use – rented from local chemists' shops.

Lying in bed can become uncomfortable after quite a short while, especially to a patient who cannot move his back without help. If he has retained the strength of his arms he can shift his position occasionally by pulling himself up with, for example, a rope ladder (7s. 9d. from the British Red Cross) to be slung over the foot rail of his bed. A more elaborate device like a spring-pole with a stirrup hand attachment (£4 4s. 0d. from Carters) can be installed beside his stronger hand in rooms between 7ft 6in and 11ft 6in high. Or a curved 'patient helper' (Carters, £9 5s. 6d. to £10 17s. 6d.) can be screwed on to the bedside rail to enable him to move about in bed and even lower himself into a wheelchair or on to a bed-pan.

Beds have already been discussed (pages 41-2) but many bed-bound people may be helped to sit up comfortably by an upholstered bedrest shaped like the back and arms of an armchair. It costs £7 19s. 0d. to £10 19s. 0d. according to size (Relyon Bedrest, from John Bell & Croyden, see Appendix for address), but can often be hired for little or nothing from local branches of the British Red Cross.

Another aid to changing positions in bed for meals, reading, TV-viewing or letter-writing is a wedge-shaped bolster which unzips in the middle, thus giving a choice of three different positions for the patient. He can lie nearly flat on it using only half the bolster, lie on a slant with it zipped together to its full depth, or stand it on its triangular base to give a firm back-rest for sitting up in bed. (Adjustapillo, by Dunlopillo, from most large stores, including John Lewis, at £2 11s. 0d. for the 2ft 6in height; £3 11s. 0d. for the 4ft 6in height.)

For other bedside equipment see Chapter 6, on Leisure.

Incontinence

Some wonderful work has been done, principally at the Stoke Mandeville Hospital, in teaching young people and children with spinal injuries to control their bowels and bladders. This is a medical problem and one to discuss with your doctor.

But at least some of the inconvenience and indignity of continued incontinence can be reduced by wearing plastic pants and disposable pads. A full list of these is available from the Disabled Living Foundation, price 2s. 6d., who have also published a comprehensive book on this – often unnecessarily – embarrassing subject: *Incontinence* by Leonora Elphick, costing 15s. 6d.

Another boon to the incontinent – and their attendants – are the non-absorbent one-way polypropylene sheets (i.e. Marathon, 22s. 6d., obtainable from chemists including John Bell & Croyden) which may enable some patients to get a dry night's rest, often for the first time in years. These sheets operate on the same principle as the candlewick: they are placed next to the patient's body and conduct any moisture to the drawsheet underneath, remaining themselves quite dry. Obviously, a waterproof plastic sheet is still necessary between the drawsheet and mattress. Nylon sheets are easy to wash and do not retain odour even after continued soiling.

Some local authorities provide special laundry services for the incontinent which will take care of sheets and nightwear.

Clothing can be adapted to the accident-prone by choosing washable fabrics, dresses with split, overlapping backs (made by Milan Gowns Ltd, 341 High Road, Wood Green, London, N22) and short under-garments to which suspenders can be fixed (made by Aldrex Ltd, Newnham, Glos.). Washing may seem an endless chore but can be cut down if separates are worn, including a wrap-around skirt which opens at the back and a top. Practical nightwear for incontinent people might be a brushed nylon nightdress with a split, overlapping back and a terry towelling dressing gown, similarly made (both from the Army & Navy Stores). Plastic shoes can be washed thoroughly. Soft furnishings made from vinyl materials can be sponged down.

Reaching aids

No arm is ever quite long enough to reach everywhere one would like: under the bed where the knitting wool has rolled, behind the fridge for dusting or to a remote corner of the ceiling for an annoying spider's web which appears to mock all efforts at cleaning.

Probably many able-bodied people would appreciate an

extra 2–3ft of arm's length, and for anyone who has difficulty in bending, stretching or reaching, a 'helping hand' will be particularly useful. This ingenious, stick-like device will pick up articles from the floor, draw the curtains and can even be used – with a duster clamped on its end – for dusting the remoter corners of one's home.

A 'helping hand' operates with a trigger at its hand-held end which causes a clamp to open and shut at its far end. A magnet will pick up pins, needles and hairpins. It is obtainable in various lengths and weights, and costs £2 to £3 from Carters.

The same principle of hand-action deferred to the other end of a stick is found in certain dressing aids (see longhandled shoehorn and stocking aid below).

Clothes

Do clothes make the man (or woman)? Reams of skilful magazine writing and exquisite photography would suggest that they do. Certainly, most invalids feel a lot better just as soon as they are allowed to get out of their pyjamas and nightwear, and women patients in hospitals are known to perk up when they are encouraged to use make-up or have a hair-do.

A pretty dress or hat may have its limitations in mending a broken heart or a smashed-up leg, but they undoubtedly have a cheering effect, no matter how marginal. The very fact of wearing everyday clothes again is like a declaration of emancipation for the bedbound. They are rejoining the world where such clothes are worn by active, useful, busy people.

But dressing in ordinary clothes again need not become an obstacle race against nearly-impossible odds presented by tight-fitting garments, fiddly fastenings or other difficulties which would have been prevented had they been properly thought about. Much can be done to adapt ordinary clothes to the physically handicapped. If necessary, it is possible to discover clothes which are specially suitable.

Dressing must be a methodical procedure, with everything necessary laid out before the start. A drawer fixed underneath the bed as already suggested can be useful for this purpose, as underwear, stockings, ties and other small but essential items can be kept in it, and taken out when required either by a helper or by the disabled patient himself in a sitting position from a stool or chair placed alongside for the purpose.

A special technique may have to be learnt. A patient with one side or limb immobile will find it easier to start the dressing operation with his 'good' side: to take it out of a jacket or coat first when undressing, to put it last into a garment when dressing so that it can do most of the necessary work for both limbs.

Fastenings may present difficulties. Obviously, large buttons or the kind of hooks and eyes used for fur coats or corsets (corset or mantle hooks and eyes) are easier to manage than small ones. Zip fasteners are more easily opened or closed if a ring or loop is attached to the tab and a chain or string can be threaded through this, especially if the zip is up the back of a dress, well beyond the reach of any but the most nimble contortionist. But the best fastener of all is versatile Velcro ribbon, made on the burr principle from two nylon lengths (see Fig. 8). This can be used on all sorts of garments which might otherwise be difficult to manage: men's trousers, brassieres, corsets, back-fastening aprons, and so on. Even ties, ready-tied in a knot, can be attached to the collar of a shirt by means of a short strip of Velcro sewn under the shirt collar on each side of the front opening. (Velcro costs 3d. per inch – 9s. per yd. – from the haberdashery departments of large stores.)

Elastic is a good and useful standby for clothes for the physically disabled too: buttons can be sewn on to a shirt or other garment with elastic thread, cuff-links can be joined in this way and elastic shoelaces can be made from ordinary narrow elastic, or bought ready-made from various shops, including Boots. Shoes with elastic side-gussets are often easier to slip on than ones with other kinds of fastenings. Elastic in the waistband of trousers and pyjamas will make these easy to pull on, and elastic straps in women's garments like brassieres or petticoats may mean that these can be slid into without adjustments to any opening (though front-fastening brassieres which can be bought or adapted may be more suitable for a woman who needs really firm support).

Probably the most difficult of all dressing problems for women is putting on stockings. Fortunately, trousers are a perfectly acceptable substitute on all but the most formal occasions,

VELCRO

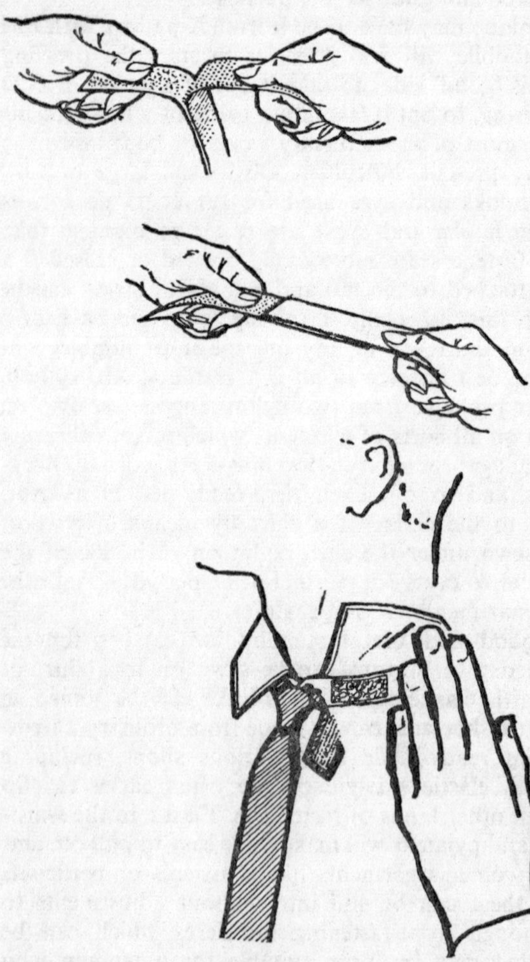

Fig. 8 Diagrams to show the use of Velcro. (From *Clothing Fastenings for the Handicapped and Disabled*, published by the Disabled Living Foundation. Drawing by Mrs B. Naylor. Velcro is made by Selectus Ltd.).

certainly for the young and middle-aged. But a 'gutter-type stocking aid' (4s. 0d. from the British Rheumatism & Arthritis Association), or a semi-circular device at the end of a stick on to which a stocking is attached by means of suspenders and then slid up the leg (£1 5s. 0d. from Carters) may be useful. A long-handled shoehorn (2s. 0d. or 4s. 6d. from the British Red Cross Society) will help with another dressing chore which troubles many elderly people.

In these days of informal dressing, no man need feel badly turned out because he chooses not to wear the waistcoat he can't manage to button, nor should a woman who can only cope with her hair by wearing it in a wide elastic band feel less than immaculate. Loose-fitting clothes are fashionable as well as sensible, and individuality can be shown by choosing a becoming colour scheme rather than tailor-made fit. The WRVS are even experimenting with an adapted man's suit which can be opened out along the external trouser seams, and can be folded round a patient, and kept in place by means of Velcro ribbon. This would certainly simplify the dressing problem for men who might otherwise spend nearly all their time in pyjamas and dressing-gowns.

For specific solutions to individual clothes problems there are two useful publications: *Clothes Fastenings for the Handicapped and Disabled*, 7s. 6d., published by the DLF, and *Help Yourselves* by P. E. Jay, E. Walker, and A. Ellison, published by Butterworths at 8s. 6d., which has a useful chapter on dressing, as well as one on personal hygiene for people whose mobility has been impaired by a stroke.

Chapter 3

Looking after physically handicapped children at home

All babies are born with certain handicaps which parents accept without question. The fact that their child can't at first see or hear very well, can't sit up, stand, walk or grip properly, adds a certain charming helplessness. Better still, the gradual acquisition of these skills, one after the other, is a matter of pride to everyone concerned: parent and child.

It is not always easy to recognize a physical handicap in a young baby, especially for new parents faced with their first child. Yet, in many cases, early diagnosis and treatment can make a substantial difference in correcting the disability, or helping a child to adjust to it. Conscientious parents can easily worry if their child does not seem to be reacting or developing as the child next door or some young cousin appears to be doing. It is worth getting a trained opinion on things which may be danger signals but may also just be part of an individual child's normal development. Regular attendance at the child's welfare clinic is one way to ensure that any baby is making reasonable progress. What may be more important, such visits will also mean that he is under constant medical supervision, so that any physical disability can be recognized and dealt with by an expert as early as possible.

It is worth getting a perspective on the kind of physical disabilities which are current: some where the numbers of afflicted children who survive are increasing, some comfortably on the decline. Out of 1,000 children, just over seven will suffer from epilepsy, over three from cerebral palsy, just over one will be blind or deaf. It does not make the individual child's plight less tragic but the relative rarity of his problem may make it easier for medical and educational services to give him their full attention. And it is surely not unreasonable to suppose that the medical skill which now enables more handicapped babies to survive will continue to research successfully into treatments for curing, or at least improving, their lot.

Handicaps affecting movement

Spastic and cerebrally palsied children

Every eight hours another spastic is born, says the Spastics Society, one of the largest and (with a budget of nearly £2 million) richest of the organizations catering for the physically handicapped. It is estimated that there are between 75–100,000 spastics in the UK suffering from greater or lesser amounts of damage to the brain which shows itself in defective movements of one sort or another, speech, vision or intellect.

All spastic babies should receive regular medical treatment as soon as their complaint has been diagnosed. That crucial first year of life when a child develops and learns so much is vital, not only for the expert treatment given but also to the way the parents support this by the way they handle their child. The parents' co-operation may be time-consuming but can mean that the child is encouraged to speak or move or hold himself upright, not only during a half-hour session at the clinic or hospital but during the longer and equally important hours he spends at home.

A useful book for parents of spastic children is *Handling the Young Cerebral Palsied Child at Home*, by Nancie R. Finnie, MCSP (former deputy principal of the Western Cerebral Palsy Centre, London, published by Heinemann Medical Books Ltd at 18s. 0d.). This will teach them to manage their spastic child patiently while he is being bathed, fed or dressed. Even quite ordinary occasions like romping with Daddy, or tidying a book-case, can be made into therapeutic occasions for a child to whom certain movements are difficult. The earlier he is encouraged to learn to use the handicapped parts of his body the more likely he is to succeed.

Certain educational theories about teaching basic movements in swimming or tennis seem to be equally valid for all children: spastics should not be allowed to get used to making movements which are definitely wrong and will prevent them from making further progress. A 'crawler' (see Fig. 9) is a useful low stool on wheels for a baby who cannot support himself on straight

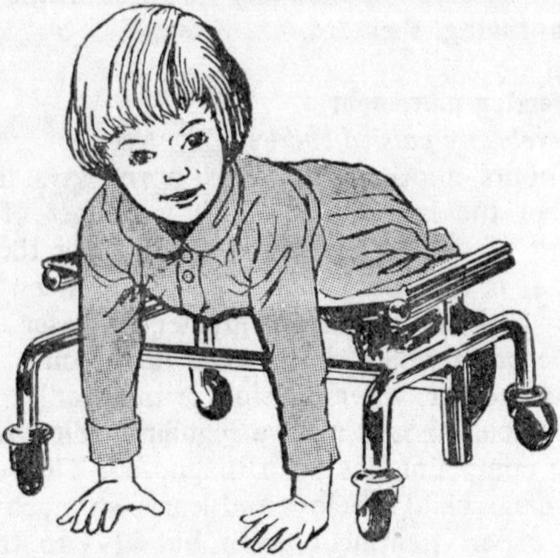

Fig. 9 Infant crawler. Designed for training young children, it is strongly constructed of steel tubing with a canvas sling covered with Vynide. The sling supports the main body weight and allows the child to take exercise. Adjustable in height from 8" to 11". (From *Equipment for Physical Medicine and Rehabilitation,* produced by J & A Carters Ltd.)

arms when trying to crawl along the floor. It will enable him to bend his hips and move his legs alternately. Children with athetoid cerebral palsy also enjoy the sense of movement given by the use of a crawler, or by special chairs, tricycles or starting rollers they can lie on while playing.

Make him feel that life has lots of interest by involving him in what you or the other children are doing: let him sit up for family meals as soon as possible even if he needs a special chair to do so, and sling a hammock or a baby swing into a doorway from which he can watch what is going on around him. Teach him to dress and undress by giving him clothes which are definitely large and therefore easier to cope with than tight ones with fiddly buttons or other fastenings (Figs. 10 and 11).

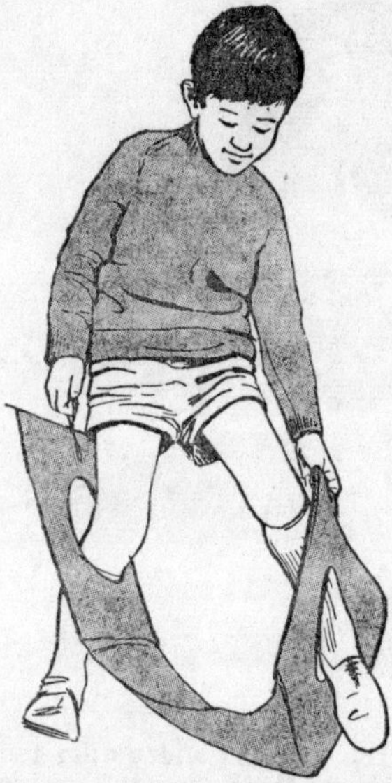

Fig. 10 A dressing aid for legs. (From the catalogue *Abbatt Developmental Toys,* produced by Paul and Marjorie Abbatt Ltd.)

Don't, on the other hand, make things too easy for him. Then he'll never realize that it's worth making an effort to get about on his own or do anything which may be difficult. If he mainly turns his head to the right, place his bed near the right-hand wall so he'll have to learn to swivel his head round to the awkward side too if he really wants to see what's happening in the rest of the room.

Spina bifida

Ten years ago nearly nine children out of ten born with spina bifida ('split spine') died within a few weeks of birth. Today, however, with new operating techniques and the insertion of a valve to drain the hydrocephalus (fluid within the brain) which

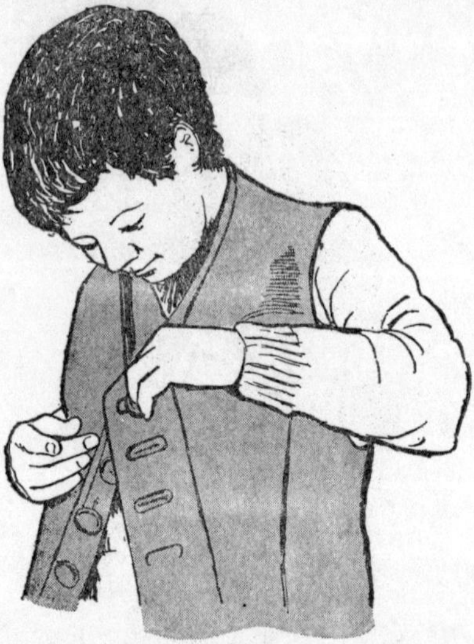

Fig. 11 Buttoning jacket. Buttons and button holes on rigid material. (From the catalogue *Abbatt Development Toys,* produced by Paul and Marjorie Abbatt Ltd.)

is so often an additional complication of this illness, more children with spina bifida survive. Over 2,500 such children are now born each year in the UK. So far, nearly 10,000 of them have survived, which means that they will soon outnumber better-known categories of physically handicapped children like, for instance, either the deaf or the blind, of school age.

Fortunately, recent advances in the treatment (surgical and orthopaedic) of spina bifida have resulted in a much better chance of normal life for children with this disability. Most of them are mentally normal and any paralysis they may have usually affects only the lower part of the body. With treatment beginning earlier and earlier in their lives – often on the very first day – more and more children will eventually walk, even if not altogether normally.

Bladder and bowel control is another problem which follows from the loss of feeling in the lower part of the body, but parents, and children over the age of six or so can be taught how to express urine or how to cope with toilet functions by means of a urine bag worn on the thigh. Certain operations, such as the production of an ileal loop, are also of assistance.

Care must be taken not to allow bladder infections to develop, especially in girls. In the case of children wearing a Holter or other valve to keep the water pressure in the brain constant and level, a headache must be treated as a danger signal that things are not working as they should. And, as with all bed- or chair-bound children, food should be balanced and no over-fond mother should be tempted to allow him to eat so much that he gets fat.

The Association for Spina Bifida and Hydrocephalus (112 City Road, London, EC1) was founded in 1966 and now has over 60 local groups. Its main aim is to meet the special needs for treatment and education of these children and to provide a meeting place for parents, nurses and doctors involved in this condition.

Limbless, including thalidomide

The soul-searing tragedy of the thalidomide babies born deformed as a result of a sedative prescribed by their doctors to their mothers in early pregnancy has perhaps obscured the fact that there have always been – and continue to be – children who are born without their full complement of healthy limbs.

Limbless children may be entirely without one or both arms or legs or they may have one or several rudimentary limbs. Thalidomide is known to have caused other deformities apart from ones affecting the limbs, but in this context of looking after such children the reference is mainly to limb deformities.

The Lady Hoare Thalidomide Appeal (78 Hamilton Terrace, London, NW8), is one of the most active of all the associations connected with specific illnesses. It employs 18 medical social workers to visit families and advise and guide parents, and has already paid out approximately £50,000 to families with thalidomide children, pending the compensation which should eventually be paid to them by the British manufacturers of the pernicious drug.

The most important single factor in home-handling of limbless children is the attitude of the parents and the extent to which they can adapt themselves and cope with the numerous difficulties.

The provision of prostheses must be planned individually to suit each child and fit in with his normal development (which, let us remember, is much like that of any other child). This means that the child will want arms and hands to reach with by the fourth month of his life, legs and feet by about the ninth. If the child's own limb, though rudimentary, is long enough to be used, it is sometimes considered best for him to learn to accommodate himself to this. Not even the best, most modern, specially powered artificial limb can provide all the learning sensations of touch and handling of even a partial limb. Another advantage of allowing a child to use his own limb, either entirely or encased in an appliance, is that this will strengthen the muscles and encourage him to further progress.

One important source of learning for babies and small children comes from what they see, and it is therefore important to help them sit up. In the case of children born without arms, artificial arms can only be fitted when they are placed in a vertical position. In the early days following the thalidomide disaster, armless as well as legless children were greatly helped by a special device known as the Chailey Flower Pot. This was used to hold a legless child from the age when a normal contemporary would be beginning to sit up independently. It then facilitated the fitting of artificial arms in this position.

As the child grows older, other problems arise which can be solved with imagination and forethought. Toys should be chosen with care, so as to amuse and instruct him without adding to his feelings of frustration. Clothes too should be the kind he will eventually be able to put on for himself in the general interest of becoming independent. Sleeves and trouser legs should be adapted to his particular disability, and tight and too-small clothing be avoided. Some limbless children may not be able to manage stairs for themselves. As they become too heavy to be carried, the family may have to consider a move to a bungalow.

Muscular dystrophy

No one seems to know for certain just how many children suffer from this disease since it is not officially notifiable, but the

Muscular Dystrophy Group (26 Borough High Street, London, SE1, and with 130 local branches) estimate that around 5,000 children suffer from the most common and severe form, and that a further 15,000 people, including young and middle-aged adults, may have similar but fortunately more benign versions.

The Duchenne type of muscular dystrophy affects mostly boys. The onset is gradual but usually starts between three and six years of age, and is often not immediately spotted because the main signs are much the kind of thing any young child may be expected to do for fun or devilment; he will fall frequently, have trouble climbing stairs, develop a peculiar waddling walk. But if the muscles in the calf of his leg are visibly enlarged too, this should be treated as a danger signal.

This disease isn't one he has caught but one he may have inherited through his mother. If she is a carrier, half her sons may be dystrophy victims and half her daughters may be carriers too. One major milestone in eradicating this disease is the fact that modern tests can spot with 90 per cent accuracy women who are carriers. Qualified medical advice should be sought by anyone who might be worried.

Muscular dystrophy is a progressive wasting disease of the voluntary muscles which makes itself known by the gradual weakening of those muscles. In time, the patient becomes confined to a wheelchair, and eventually to bed. Every care should be taken to delay the course of the illness by encouraging the child to keep using his weakening muscles. Swimming is an activity which he can share with the rest of the family. If possible, he should get an education which teaches him to make use of his full intelligence so as to stand him in good stead when physical activities are beyond him.

While doctors and research workers are hoping to solve the challenge of muscular dystrophy, parents of afflicted boys must do what they can to ensure that their children continue to lead as full and active a life as possible for as long as they can.

One recommendation is to avoid a diet which will cause the child to put on too much weight. Over-weight is always a danger, especially to children who are bedbound. Bronchitis is sometimes dangerous for dystrophic children because the chest muscles may be too weak to cough properly.

Another problem common to this disease is that the feet eventually become too deformed for ordinary footwear. Slipper-sox, those knitted calf-length socks with a soft slipper sole originally evolved for après-ski wear, are recommended at this stage.

Other handicaps

Blindness

It is obviously tempting to over-protect a blind baby from the large world he can't see. But although he must not be allowed to hurt himself unnecessarily, or get frightened, he must be guided and stimulated to independence, just like other children.

Like them, he will need to develop an interest in toys, to be toilet-trained and to be taught to feed himself. Get him to know about the things he can't see: the rattle, the toothbrush, the pot (and later, the lavatory), the spoon, plate and mug by letting him feel them when they're clean.

Accomplishments like these will give him confidence and make his life more interesting too. Read to him from books and tell him about the picture 'on this page' (let him feel it) – 'teddy is playing with his tricycle' – and try to relate what you are talking about to the things he knows about: toys, people, homes and so on. He'll depend on you for many of his experiences.

Almost more than other children, a blind child who is otherwise fit and well will need to develop self-confidence and independence. Make sure he gets exercise by taking him for walks whenever possible and teach him to ride a tricycle in some safe spot where he can bump into the edges of the grass or the side of a building to know where he is. Learning to swim is fun for him, and he'll be able to enjoy using a gym, to climb a rope, to dance and listen to music. Try to keep him busy and interested so that he won't develop the idle and unsightly 'habit movements' of many bored blind children.

Don't hand him a rattle or toy whenever he seems to be at a loose end. Teach him to find his own toys where they are kept: in a corner of his pram or play-pen at first, then later in a special box or drawer. Try and set aside one room for his own use, so he can gain confidence in his ability to find things for himself.

As his parent, you'll have to become very methodical and

far-sighted. Always put his things where they belong and shut doors of rooms he's not supposed to get out of. Once he's got to know the lay-out of his own room, don't change it without telling him and taking him round first. You don't want him roaming the house in search of some much-loved baby-chair or cot you've got rid of. Tell him he's a big boy now and ready for a large bed like the one used by his big brother or the boy across the road. Be imaginative about his difficulties. Teach him to feel doors for their handles and to open them carefully so as not to bang himself, and to approach chests or cupboards searching for the handles with which he can pull out the drawers. You can't abolish the stairs so you must teach him to negotiate them, feet first, and sliding down on his tummy. Later, he'll be ready for the bannisters and he'll learn to tell where he is from the sound of his footsteps. A loud-ticking clock in a room will help him find his way about and a ball with a bell is easier to retrieve when lost. Often, he'll have to be stimulated into playing with something he can't see anyone else doing: pushing a train about or fitting pegs into a pattern or, later, playing solitaire or chess. A push-toy will encourage him to walk and has the added advantage of bumping into things before he does.

The Royal National Institute for the Blind (224/8 Great Portland Street, London, W1) has a parents' unit to advise parents of blind children how to make the best of their ability and how to make full use of formal education. The Social Welfare Officer who visits blind children as part of the Local Authority's Blind Welfare Scheme should also be able to provide guidance, especially when she knows the child and the rest of the family.

From five to sixteen, formal education is compulsory. Most blind children go to special schools, usually as boarders, or to special classes in ordinary schools where braille is used for reading and writing and other special apparatus is employed for learning. Boarding schools are particularly useful because blind children must not only learn the usual academic subjects but a whole technique of living as well. Later they can transfer to one or two residential grammar schools at eleven, though in the case of children under six and a half, or after 'O' levels, blind children from normal loving homes can share educational facilities with other, normal children.

Blind students can and do go to universities and for further training. Blind people have trained to become lawyers, computer programmers, social welfare workers, teachers, physiotherapists, shorthand-typists, telephonists, etc., but their training and employment will need to be decided upon in full knowledge of all the facts by the welfare and educational services in consultation with parents at least a year before they leave school.

The National Library Service for the Blind (see Appendix for address) provides books for blind and partially-sighted children as well as for adults. Special magazines for children in various age groups between five and six and teenagers are published by the RNIB and the Scottish Braille Press, Edinburgh. Blind students on university courses can have textbooks specially taped for them by the British Talking Book Service for the Blind (Mount Pleasant, Wembley, Middx). Recordings are free of charge but the machine for them must be rented for £3 0s. 0d. per annum.

Deaf children (including those with partial hearing)

It must already be obvious how difficult it is to classify children, or indeed people, like stamps. Certainly, deaf children do not easily fall into one or other category: a child who becomes deaf after he has learnt to speak has only lost one sense (albeit a very important one), whereas a child deaf from birth will also be without speech and has therefore two major problems. Another important sub-group are the 250 or so deaf and blind rubella children whose handicap results from the fact that their mothers had German measles during the one to three months after they had been conceived and many of whom, therefore, suffer from two handicaps, although one may be slighter than the other.

Education is very important for all deaf children. They are only too easily considered stupid or even subnormal when their main learning difficulty is that they can't hear. The earlier a child's deafness can be diagnosed the better for him, especially as this gives him a chance of getting used to a hearing aid, and enables him to leave his own shut-off loneliness and communicate with other people; 8–10 months' old babies are not considered too young for a hearing aid. As he gets older, an identity disc is useful in case he gets lost and can't tell anyone his name and address.

Mothers and fathers of deaf children have a very special problem. Normal children learn to speak during the pre-school period, and it is most important to take advantage of these precious learning years to make the most of what residual hearing your child has.

Give your child as much listening practice as possible by talking to him and playing with him. He must be made to realize by touch and by effect, if nothing else, that there are sounds and that they differ. Speak to him as you would to the other children in the family or to the household pet, to show him that speech is important, that it means love and affection, or food ('would you like some more dessert?') or discipline ('don't pull the tablecloth off the table!').

Parents cannot be expected to assume the role of special teacher to the deaf. But they should make sure that the precise nature of their child's deafness is expertly diagnosed. He will probably need a hearing aid, and also speech therapy, in order, if at all possible, to grasp 'oral communication', i.e. speech. Sign language and finger spelling is definitely a second-best.

The National Deaf Children's Society (31 Gloucester Place, London, W1H 4EA) publishes in its annual report a complete list, with maps, of all day schools, boarding schools (including ones taking weekly boarders), and partially hearing units attached to ordinary schools. The National Association for Deaf, Blind and Rubella Children (61, Senneleys Park Road, Northfield, Birmingham 31) is particularly interested in special education units for these children. Finally, there is one organization which particularly welcomes partially hearing school-leavers, the British Association of the Hard of Hearing, Hon. Secretary, C. H. Mardell, Briarfield, Syke Ings, Iver, Bucks.

Epilepsy

One major difference between epilepsy and the other physical handicaps discussed in this chapter is the fact that there is no overwhelmingly pressing need for early diagnosis which – in all the other sections discussed – would give the young sufferer a better chance of being cured or adjusting to his disability by all that doctors and physiotherapists can do for him.

Epilepsy is like an electrical storm in the brain which disturbs its smooth and efficient functioning. It can take many forms, ranging from a brief and often practically unnoticeable 'absence' when the patient may look blank or twitch slightly, and be unable to see or hear for a few seconds (the *petit mal*) to longer periods of unconsciousness when he may fall to the ground and lose consciousness, roll his eyes, twitch, maybe froth at the mouth, and soil himself (*grand mal*).

The main problem of epilepsy is that its occurrence is entirely unpredictable, although drugs can usually keep it under control. The violence of the seizures can be greatly reduced or even entirely eliminated in this way. But the child should be under regular medical supervision, at least initially, until his parents and teachers and, later, he himself, have been taught what to do. With modern methods of treatment, most epileptics are now able to lead a normal life, but it will take some years before your doctor can predict with confidence what course your child's illness is taking.

Most epileptic children can participate in sports, but cycling and climbing are not recommended. A child who gets a few seconds' warning of an impending *grand mal* attack in the shape of an 'aura' may even be able to swim, provided he makes sure to remove himself to a place of safety in time. Working with workshop tools which may be potentially dangerous during a fit is also not recommended, although it is said that utter absorption in the job at hand seems to inhibit the likelihood of an attack. Grown-up epileptics too have to bear this risk in mind: certain jobs which involve driving a truck or working on potentially dangerous machines or being responsible for the safety of others are never considered suitable for epileptics.

The British Epilepsy Association (3–6 Alfred Place, London, WC1) is trying to fill many of the gaps still left in the State and local authority services for the epileptic, including especially information and advice, and an improvement in public understanding, as well as more research into its causes.

Cystic fibrosis

Another children's disease which can now be treated – if not yet cured – is a chronic disorder of the mucus secreting glands in which abnormally sticky mucus can affect the child's lungs and digestion.

About 400 new cases occur in the UK each year. In a baby the symptoms are foul-smelling stools, a cough which is unusual for one of such tender age, and an inability to gain weight. Medical advice and skilled treatment from a physiotherapist will be essential, especially at first, until the routine is fully established. Then good home care can make all the difference to his future.

The main problem for parents will be to help the child make the best use of his lungs and keep them clear and undamaged by regular breathing exercises. In the case of a baby or for a very young child this means giving percussion to the chest and postural drainage to stimulate coughing. The Cystic Fibrosis Research Trust (Stuart House, 1 Tudor Street, London, EC4) publishes a booklet, *Postural Drainage at Home* by Diana Gaskell, MCSP, superintending physiotherapist, explaining in words and photographs how this can be done by parents at home without special equipment.

When the child is older he will eventually have learnt from experience that two to three daily sessions of coughing in a private place where he can't be overheard by possibly mocking playmates will enable him to work and play happily the rest of the time without a perpetual cough.

Nowadays, children with cystic fibrosis can grow up and have a normal home and school life, provided they get proper attention, medication, and that their lungs remain undamaged. Their diet also needs careful supervision. They must be given plenty of proteins and vitamins because their bodies are not able to absorb all the food they eat.

Speech impairment

Among the other physical handicaps we've been considering in this chapter, a mere speech impairment may seem relatively trivial. But a child who can't speak at all or insufficiently clearly to be understood is deprived of an essential human ability. He is actually or virtually dumb. So it's definitely worth making the effort to do everything possible to put this right.

Treatment for this condition depends to some extent on its cause: was the child born deaf or with impaired hearing? With a deformity like a cleft palate? Does he suffer from cerebral palsy? Is he mentally retarded? Are emotional difficulties inhibiting him? So if your child is not saying a few words at the age of two, and certainly if he's still babbling unintelligibly by the time he's three, take him to the clinic to have him investigated. He may well need the attention of a speech therapist who will teach him from her technical understanding of his particular difficulties. Don't be tempted to find one without specialist help.

The parents' contribution towards teaching their child to speak is mainly patience and perseverance. They must reinforce the speech therapist's teaching by talking frequently to their child, speaking slowly and clearly, making sure he understands what they say. They must give him every opportunity to speak by asking him questions and waiting patiently for his answer. If his speech is so indistinct that they're not sure they've really understood him, they must repeat what they think he said and get him to confirm or deny it.

Constant noise and distraction is an enemy of the concentration he will need to speak. Turn the television set off or make use of some programme your child has been watching by talking about it, asking him: Have you ever seen a dog (car, aeroplane, house, etc.) like that before? How old do you think he is? Would you like to visit New York (the country, the zoo, etc.)?

Take time to read to your child, preferably when you're alone together, sitting him on your knee so you can look at the pictures in the book together, and get him to repeat names or phrases after you or ask him questions about the story. If the other children like to interrupt and override the brother or sister with speech difficulties, tell them to be quiet, sending them out of the room if necessary. Many a younger child never gets a chance to open his mouth when the older ones are there, determined to have their say *first*.

Multiple handicaps

Among the many physically handicapped who can be helped in so many ingenious ways, the plight of the child with multiple handicaps is often the most pitiable. He may suffer only a mild degree of each particular disability, but this may mean that assessment and treatment of his actual capacities and problems is that much more difficult to make. Unfortunately, the physiotherapist who can help him to move is not at the same time a speech therapist who can help him to speak. If he is a spastic child, it may be difficult to judge whether he does not react to stimuli because his brain is impaired or because he is also deaf.

Often, such children are educationally subnormal. This is so vast a problem as to be beyond the scope of a book like this which centres on physical disability. Many others are emotionally maladjusted, which is probably only too easily understood when one thinks of the special problems all physically handicapped children have to face as they grow up.

Most experts agree that treatments for multiple handicaps have to be tackled one at a time: fundamental ones like, for instance, heart surgery, before less urgent ones like audiometry (assessment of hearing). But if one particular disability is likely to respond to *early* treatment, then that obviously takes priority, especially if, as a result, a child with several handicaps may become a child with only one which can then be treated as such.

A careful balance must be struck between a child's educational and medical (or surgical) needs. Uninterrupted schooling is most important to all children. It is better to attend to the child's medical needs before seven or eight if this is likely to allow the young patient a clear period from then until fifteen or sixteen rather than to break up his education with repeated spells of hospital treatment. Once off the educational bus (or pressure cooker?) getting on again becomes more difficult, not only because so much has been missed but also because the habit of school learning has to be re-started.

If one of the child's physical disabilities is a sensory one like blindness or deafness, the training for this should take precedence at home and at school over any other treatment he may need. This is his only chance of ever being able to follow normal education, even with other physically handicapped children.

Children suffering from multiple handicaps can come into so

many varied categories of disability, such as blindness, deafness, lack of speech, asthma or epilepsy, cerebral palsy or other troubles, that it would be impossible to mention each one and equally impossible to cater for each combination separately. Attendance at special care units or special boarding schools for children with multiple handicaps is usually found to be the best possible way to educate such children to some degree of independence, not only in school and in academic attainments but also in looking after themselves. Often, a sheltered workshop is considered to provide a more suitable working environment for their adult lives than complete independence, though some lucky children with unusual gifts and persistence may be able to break out beyond this.

Parents' attitudes and encouragement

No conscientious parent takes parenthood altogether lightly. But the parents of a child with a physical handicap bear a specially heavy responsibility. Their main difficulty is to remember that he is primarily a child, then someone who will have to learn to live like other children, and finally still a physically handicapped person who will grow up, and have to live with his disability. Their very natural first instinct may be to over-protect him.

It may be a cliché to talk about a problem shared being a problem halved, but sayings are not necessarily untrue because they are too often used glibly. Certainly, it's essential for *both* parents to face their child's problem realistically, and discuss it quite frankly with one another.

Later on their child too will be helped by a frank discussion of his handicap. This helps him to face his future and gain some idea of how he will be able to live when he grows up.

One of the unnecessary difficulties experienced by many parents of physically handicapped children is a feeling of guilt, especially if the child's handicap has evidently become worse as a result of their failure to take him to the doctor in time, or even more so if he has become physically disabled as the result of an accident or illness from which they feel they should have protected him. So they hide him away, which helps nobody, instead of facing the fact that no one – no matter how loving and conscientious – can protect anyone else from all the hazards of living – certainly not without endangering the child's normal desire for independence as he gets older.

The problem is not theirs alone: it is a national one. A handicapped child who has been trained to live independently and educated to earn his own living is not only happier in himself but is also a net gain to the whole community.

It may be understandable that the mother of a spastic child is simply too tired from the inevitable strain of looking after him to avail herself of all the advice and help she could get if she only asked for it, especially if she has other children too. Moreover, parents of physically handicapped children sometimes feel – not altogether without justification – that they have become to some extent handicapped themselves. They cannot do the things which other families do: go on holiday, maybe, or have a picnic in the park or send him round to the grocer for a pound of sugar.

Some of these hesitations are justified, but some are not. Physically handicapped children certainly complicate outings, but with a little extra arrangement an outing to a circus or even a holiday in a recommended hotel, camp or caravan site is entirely possible. Even inquisitive neighbours or tactless inquirers eventually learn to accept a physically handicapped child and take him for granted. Your child, for his part, must get to know people of all sorts, and learn to get on with them.

Too often it is as though the child's physical handicap exerts a handicapping effect on his whole family: parents, brothers and sisters, grandparents, even aunts and uncles. This attitude may be understandable when you remember how much extra care and attention the child needs, with all the endlessly repetitive daily details of washing and dressing, toilet-training, eating, playing, walking, and so on, and how little apparent progress there often is to show for all the painstaking, loving attention which is lavished on him, but it is all the same positively damaging to the innocent young originator who is meant to be shielded from harm.

Like any other child, the physically handicapped may be clever or dull, artistic or musical, good with his hands or mechanically-minded, untidy, noisy, inattentive, loving, irritating – in fact, altogether human. Given ordinary health in other respects he will grow up and will therefore have to be trained to adjust to the world about him if he is not to be shoved aside by the relentless onward march of his peers in the nursery, and later at school, at work or at play.

The parents' role is to train their child, any child, able-bodied or physically handicapped, to the activities of daily living, to teach him self-discipline, to give him a sense of security by loving him, and a sense of self-confidence by providing him with the opportunity to play and to widen his experience of life to the extent that he is able to accept it.

Toys

Play is an important learning activity for all children, and of even more vital importance to the physically handicapped whose activities and learning opportunities are necessarily more limited. Good toys will help them to learn many things about space, proportion, balance, etc. which more active children may already have discovered for themselves. What's more, satisfying play sessions will help them develop, adjust to other people, including children, and keep them quiet and concentrated for varying periods.

Choose your child's toys carefully, making sure that he can enjoy playing and learning in this way and try to eliminate any which are likely to be unduly frustrating: i.e. too fiddly, too easily breakable or frankly beyond his age group or skill. Be imaginative about play equipment. At Chailey Heritage an armless thalidomide child of five spent happy hours rocking himself in a plastic baby rocker which looked like something out of space fiction and had originally been designed for too-energetic toddlers; and the pupils of Wanstead High School have ingeniously adapted tricycles to enable children who can't walk to get about under their own steam. A walking tricycle can be bought from Carters (see Appendix for address) and will encourage children with weak limbs to get about and exercise them.

A visit to a large toy shop or a local play group of his contemporaries may give you all sorts of ideas to follow up for your child: bowls or boxes in which to keep beads so that they don't roll away, water-play with beakers over a basin, modelling with clay, plasticine or flour and water, and music making. Mental stimulation is every bit as important as having fun and usually far more satisfying in the long run. Remind him to make a cake or maybe a banana when he's modelling, to pretend he's shampooing each finger separately when he's washing his hands, to beat time to music on the radio.

Not that all toys need be educational. Dolls and stuffed animals have a function too: every child needs something to love and cuddle and dream over. Presumably most parents of home-bound young children know about the television and radio programmes especially aimed at this age group: *Play School*, *Watch with Mother*, *Listen with Mother*, *Jackanory* and so on. These don't merely help a young child to pass the time, but often stimulate the imagination and prod them into activities like collecting, painting, cutting out, much as a good nursery teacher would.

A stimulating selection of toys specially designed to simplify the understanding of elementary skills like sorting, selecting, copying, assembling, drawing, building, counting and dressing for handicapped children is on sale in the Abbatt Developmental Toys range by Paul and Marjorie Abbatt Ltd. Write to them at PO Box 57, High Wycombe, Bucks, for a catalogue and price-list. The toys are also usually on view in the basement of their shop at 94 Wimpole Street, London, W1. They go beyond learning activities to include also dressing aids as well as toys like large mosaic pattern pieces to encourage group activities among children who may have become solitary-minded as a result of their disability. Handicapped children often lack the opportunity to meet other people and may not have had the chance to develop a talent or an inclination to play together.

A useful book giving detailed instructions on how to set about teaching handicapped children of pre-school and school age to use play material with a view to acquiring basic skills like dressing themselves, cutting out, sewing, building and even reading is *Practical Training for the Severely Handicapped Child* by Milan Morgenstern, Helen Low-Beer and Franz Morgenstern (published by Heinemann Medical Books at 21s. 0d., and obtainable through the Spastics Society).

Although mainly intended for teachers and therapists of mentally handicapped children, this book describes how to avoid frustrations with equipment, like the recalcitrant scissors which won't open again once shut, or how to concentrate attention on one passage of reading material. These problems can happen to any child and can make him feel unnecessarily inadequate and incapable.

Some toys can be specially adapted to the needs of the child, like ping-pong bats with thickened handles, or go-karts with padded and extended bumpers, tricycles with pedals or specially weighted push-toys to help him walk without risk of going too fast. Specially chosen toys are remedial for children with certain handicaps: a yoyo for a stiff shoulder, dart-throwing to develop the elbow, or threading wooden rings together on a central stick to make a figure on a pyramid for developing the hand and fingers. There is unsuspected therapy too in all sorts of quite ordinary toys like plastic construction kits, question and answer sets, tiddlywinks, pick-up sticks, and so on. Weighted dolls' prams or baby walkers filled with bricks are a great enticement and help to children with walking difficulties.

Other effective toys with therapeutic properties are the puppets made for a girl with lazy fists by the pupils of Wanstead High School on their Aid for the Disabled Project. Skater boards to slide about on will help spina bifida children to strengthen their shoulders and arms so that they can use crutches and wheelchairs later on.

Important as toys are to a child's – any child's – development, care should be taken not to burden him with things he can't do yet, or may even never be able to do. There's no point in making him feel more frustrated than he does already because the jig-saw puzzle is too difficult or because he can't read the letters on a set of building bricks. Let him graduate to more complicated toys, to gymnastic apparatus, to scissors or paints or an abacus when he's ready. Then he'll gain confidence which will in turn encourage him to make further progress.

Toy libraries

Unfortunately, good toys are often expensive. Many parents who are already faced with the expense of bringing up a child needing extra attention and care, thus depriving the mother of a chance of earning money, may not be in a position to spend a great deal of money on toys and play equipment. One solution is to join a toy library (or to start one, if there isn't one in your area).

The first toy library in the UK was sponsored by the Enfield Society for Mentally Handicapped Children, but now it also has borrowers who are spastic, thalidomide, autistic and aphasic. It cuts across the exclusiveness of societies catering for one physical handicap rather than another, and has not only brought together parents with similar problems but given their children a chance of meeting one another and playing together.

A local toy library can be started on as little as £20 and works in the expected manner of any library, with a nominal monthly borrowing fee and strict book-keeping control of borrowed goods. Special educational toys from school suppliers and special sources can usually be obtained, often at a discount. It is best to concentrate on toys which will develop the young borrower's skills.

For information and a toy index of items for inclusion write to: The Organizer, Noak's Ark Toy Libraries, 21 Gentleman's Row, Enfield, Middlesex, sending a 4d. stamp.

Recreation

Leisure and sports facilities for physically handicapped children are even more vital than for their able-bodied brothers and sisters. They are not merely a relief from boredom and tension but fill a special educational and social need. At last, an interest a disabled brother or sister has of his own.

The Information Service for the Disabled (Vincent House, Vincent Square, London, SW1) will suggest holiday recreations and amusements to suit individual and local requirements from a wide range. Admittedly, provision varies in different parts of the country but their suggestions include sports (such as golf, swimming, pony riding, fishing and sailing), games (for instance, table tennis, croquet, archery, shooting, snooker and billiards), crafts and hobbies (like music, gardening, cooking, dressmaking, dressing up, and play-reading), and various other pastimes, all of which have proved successful with other children.

Physically handicapped children can become scouts and guides, cub scouts and brownies, either in ordinary packs with able-bodied children or in extension groups run in hospitals or special schools. Generally speaking it is thought that children who are not severely handicapped are encouraged by mixing with able-bodied children. For more specific information for boys, write to the Headquarters Commissioner, Extension Activities, The Scout Association, 25 Buckingham Palace Road, London, SW1. Girls are recommended to contact their nearest local pack or to ask the pack leader for the name of their local Extension Adviser. They also have 'post units' for home-bound children who can have 'meetings' by means of sending composite scrap-books, with occasional actual get-togethers as and when these can be managed.

Teenagers and young people up to twenty-five can join the PHAB (i.e. clubs consisting of PHysically handicapped and ABle-bodied). Write to the National Association of Youth Clubs (30 Devonshire Street, London, W1) for the address of 22 such clubs in England, Wales and N. Ireland. The aim here is a two-way integration between the young disabled and their able-bodied contempories who may never have given disablement much thought before.

Many physically handicapped children attend special boarding schools, and may therefore be very glad to spend their holidays at home with the families they see relatively rarely. Even then, they should not be allowed to feel that they are suspended in a temporary vacuum between two periods of normal activities. They should be encouraged to spend their holidays happily. Lady Allen of Hurtwood has already sponsored three Holiday Clubs for Handicapped Children and is now engaged on a plan for an Adventure Club for such children.

Help from medical services and voluntary societies

Although the National Health Service provides medical and therapeutic care for the physically handicapped in all parts of the UK, the organization of these services varies from one area to another.

As far as the medical problems are concerned, your GP, paediatrician or child welfare clinic should be the essential starting point. From them you should be able to find out what your child's special needs are, and where they can be attended to. Local facilities for physiotherapy, remedial exercises, special teaching, provision of surgical appliances vary. Even a skilled doctor with a large practice may not have come across many children suffering from one particular kind of physical handicap such as, for example, a blind baby or a limbless child, before. What he will know is the point of contact inside your local authority's welfare services or at the nearest hospital where specialist services can be obtained.

One comfort about a child who is physically handicapped from birth – or even merely at risk of handicap as a result of a difficult birth or a previous illness of his mother – is that he will usually be under medical supervision from the start and that his parents will therefore get help and advice on how to cope with his particular physical and development problems. In most areas the local authority operates a special register for such children from birth or arrival in the area, and this means that immediate treatment can be given to, say, the deaf or the spastic at an age when it will do most good.

Sometimes the points on which you require guidance may be practical ones, too down-to-earth and petty to bother the doctor with. A health visitor may be able to discuss the preparations of your child's special diet with you in your own home. The district nurse may call to show you how best to hold your handicapped baby in his bath. Even the local Citizens Advice Bureau may be able to tell you what special services for physically handicapped children are available locally: home teachers, nursery schools, holiday relief or transport to take the young patient to hospital if necessary.

The point at which medical problems become ones of every-day living may lie somewhere between being told that your child needs fresh air and exercise, and not knowing what kind of exercise he is capable of; between a recommendation to take him for audiometric assessment, and not knowing where to leave the other children when you go; between giving him all the attention he needs and still being fair to the rest of the family, especially when it's a matter of holidays, moving house, or enabling mother to get out of the house occasionally.

Is there anyone to whom all these problems can be taken? One way to discover that you are not alone in your predicament is to join the appropriate association of parents whose children suffer from the same or a similar handicap (see list on pages 130-7).

You may well find that you are in fact much luckier than many others whose children are more severely disabled than yours. Another benefit from membership of such an organization is access to all the useful information they have amassed as a result of their personal experience about just the kind of subjects which worry you. Even though most of the headquarter offices of these associations are in London or Southern England there may be local branches in other parts of the country. If not, they can still usually provide names and addresses of local doctors, medical social workers and other specialists in your child's disability whom you can then contact direct.

Some of the practical solutions which have been tried and found to be successful are ingenious, as in the case of certain children – spastics, or without speech from some other cause – who have been taught to overcome their communication difficulties in some way other than speech. One aphasic (i.e. speechless) six-year-old was taught to use an electronic typewriter. Other children may learn to express themselves, and to overcome the frustration of being set apart, by writing or painting, or in pantomime.

If your child doesn't really seem to fit properly into any of the categories for which associations already exist it may be worth discussing with your doctor or the hospital or the National Fund for Research into Crippling Diseases (see Appendix for address) whether his case is sufficiently frequently duplicated to start another organization. This can be done in various ways, locally or on a national scale. So far, one of the most successful ways seems to have been through a letter to the Woman's Page *The Guardian*, which has launched so many invaluable national organizations.

One way to circumvent a wearisome search round existing agencies to discover one which fits your child's case is to contact the Invalid Children's Aid Association (see Appendix for address), who will give advice and help to individual parents of handicapped children. In London and the Home Counties, the ICAA has a family case-work service which includes regular visits from social workers who can provide guidance and practical aid. Outside this area they will put families in touch with someone in their own locality who can help, working usually through local authorities and other voluntary associations.

The ICAA runs schools and centres for handicaps not otherwise catered for by anyone. These include two schools providing a complete education for boys with chronic asthma and a school for intelligent children with speech and language difficulties.

Another central information service is the National Bureau for Co-operation in Child Care, where an accepted body of knowledge on the welfare, education and treatment of children (normal as well as handicapped) is being collected.

Arrangements for schooling

Should physically handicapped children go to a special school or to an ordinary one?

The experts' answer seems to be unequivocally in favour of ordinary schools. 'There is,' say the organizers of Action for the Crippled Child, 'no solution to be found in the separation of the disabled from the able-bodied. The disabled must live in society side by side and at ease with the able-bodied, and the responsibility of those who are concerned for the disabled is to make this two-way acceptance possible.'

In any case, one or two individuals can always be imperceptibly absorbed into a group, whether they are different in looks, race, speech or other feature. During World War II evacuee children from towns even found this reaction among the children in the reception areas: one or two could be integrated, ten to fifteen constituted a foreign community to be isolated and shunned. In youth clubs, too, a group of physically handicapped children all joining the same club tend to stick together and derive little benefit from the community: it is easier for one or two such children to be absorbed in a group. In bringing up a physically handicapped child, as in so many other educational enterprises, it's best to start off as you mean to go on. The ability to share every-day activities with normal children will be invaluable to him as he grows up, trains for a career, plans his future life, including work and maybe marriage.

Obviously, the education a physically handicapped child gets must be suited to his particular needs beyond the considerations meted out to his normal contemporaries. As his physical handicap may rule out several aspects of school, and may equally debar him later in life from certain active jobs requiring principally strength and dexterity, his chances of a worthwhile and satisfying future will be greatly enhanced by developing those things he *can* do, using his hands, his brain and his academic talents. He should be encouraged to focus his interests on those academic or bookish subjects at which he can do at least as well as normal children, even if the going seems hard, especially at first.

Compulsory schooling in the UK starts at the age of five, but it has been found that many physically handicapped children benefit particularly from the skills and adjustments they learn to make at nursery school age. It's easier for small children to integrate with normal children than it would be later on. If they're lucky, and well-taught, theirs is the world they'll grow up into.

Increasingly local authorities are now fitting physically handicapped children into nursery or special play groups where their needs – especially in the case of the deaf and blind children – can be catered for by specially trained teachers. If no such special nursery group is available locally, a physically handicapped child will often qualify as a priority case for an ordinary one. But a deaf child will need special auditory training from a very early age – lip-reading is useful but a lot less important – so he may have to have at least part of his education in a special unit where he can be taught skills of hearing and speaking which other children take for granted. Often, these units are attached to a normal school. Many areas now also employ special peripatetic teachers of the deaf who can visit children regularly in their homes as well as at school or clinics.

Among the many other continual distractions of family life, many parents defer decisions about their child's schooling until just before the fifth birthday, especially if they are basically a little afraid of the problem. However, education is too continuous a process to be considered as something which only happens at school during three terms a year, and at certain hours each weekday.

Pre-school nursery age education can be of immense help to physically handicapped children. If no local facilities exist, it may be worth discussing your child's case with one of the organizations concerned with his kind of handicap. Sometimes they may be able to provide parents with suggestions and advice on how to teach their child to cope with and overcome his problems. In other cases, as with blind children, residential schooling may be recommended, often starting before normal school age.

The important fact to bear in mind is that local education authorities are normally willing to consider a child even well before he approaches his fifth birthday, especially in the case of a handicapped child whose educational future can already be mapped out and routed through his special hurdles by the time he is two or three years old. For children with cerebral palsy, the Spastics Society's Family Services Assessment Centre (see also page 102) will provide a special test of his all-round potential. The local education authority will usually pay for this valuable service. Other handicapped children below school age can be sent for educational assessments by the GP or clinic, certainly by the time they are three.

The choice of school is always important, though for a physically handicapped child there is always the extra problem of making sure that his intellectual potential has been correctly assessed, even if his disability possibly precludes him from expressing himself as freely as his able-bodied contemporaries.

Generally speaking, an ordinary school is the kind to aim for, especially for a child who is lively and of at least average intelligence, though sometimes special arrangements may have to be made for him in the provision of a downstairs classroom, the use of a WC and some help from the school nurse or matron. Most epileptic children, for instance, are able to attend normal schools and profit from the teaching they receive there, as well as from the company of normal children. Sometimes a physically handicapped child can follow lessons at his desk but sitting in his own wheelchair.

But if the local school is unable or unwilling to accept your child, a day school for physically handicapped children may be the next kind to try for. These schools usually collect their pupils each day and return them to their homes in the afternoon.

Finally, there are the special residential boarding schools, some of them specializing in pupils suffering from one or other physical handicap which can be suggested to you by your local education authority or selected from a list of 'Special Schools for Handicapped Pupils' (Department of Education and Science, List 42), which can be consulted at your local library. Blind pupils and partially sighted, deaf and partially hearing, epileptic, delicate and physically handicapped, pupils suffering from a speech defect, or from more than one handicap, are all catered for at all levels of intelligence, including university entrance qualifications.

Independent schools recognized as efficient for which fees are paid either by parents or local authorities also accept physically handicapped children (List 70). For normally intelligent children with speech difficulties due to brain damage or other physical causes, the Invalid Children's Aid Association runs schools, and there are also special boarding schools for children suffering from asthma. With the virtual disappearance of children suffering from polio, there are now more places available at special residential schools for children suffering from spina bifida. Usually, most special schools are full to capacity, so that places are limited and should be applied for as early as possible, either direct to the local Medical Officer of Health or through the local Education Authority. Sometimes a limited period at a special school is all that is required during the course of a child's education.

Boarding school education has a special educational function – as well as the usual academic one – of teaching a child to stand on his own feet (metaphorically speaking, in this context!) and become self-reliant when he is away from his parents and the familiar framework of his own home. This ability to live independently may be of special value to the school leaver when he considers further career training or university, which will almost certainly require him to live away from home.

During the actual boarding period, however, parents should take great care to keep a close loving link with their child at school. Sometimes weekly boarding is possible, This seems to comprise the best – as well, it is sometimes said, as the worst! – features of both kinds of school. But regular letters and visits are one way to ensure your child retains his place in the family, especially if he has brothers or sisters who remain always with you. His holidays should be carefully planned so that he does not feel excluded because he has had no opportunity to make friends or activities of his own at home.

Chapter 4

Getting round and about

Personal mobility has been called 'one of the most precious achievements of modern civilization' – not by a physically handicapped person, staring wistfully out of his cell window, but by an Official White Paper on Public Transport and Traffic.

Certainly, getting out of one's house and into the street or park, to the office, the shops, to Church or the theatre, can be a very important source of comfort and happiness. Nor is this a contradiction of everything which has been said about the joys of living at home rather than in an institution where everything, including joint outings, can be taken care of. Even a congenial, well-loved home is only a base and a background. It should not be allowed to become a prison.

The ability to go out and get about is part of normal modern living and therefore a very natural aim for any physically handicapped person. It is essential for anyone who wants to follow a profession or do a job or train for one either on leaving school or after an accident or illness which necessitates a change of occupation. Even housewives or people whose work can be done at home (teachers, writers, artists, men running their own business, etc.) benefit from regular outings. They're stimulating and healthy, too.

Fortunately, not every physically disabled person is rendered immobile by his condition, although he is at least likely to be slowed up by it. Elderly people usually learn to come to terms with this problem too, and to allow themselves more time for errands or outings than they used to in the days when they could more easily cope with last-minute alterations to their time schedule in the shape of some shopping to do in the lunch-hour from the office, queuing for tickets to some popular play or football match, or dropping in on a friend.

Much can be done by careful planning and forethought. Often all that is necessary is a telephone call to ascertain beforehand whether the shop stocks a certain product, whether there's a seat available from the box office, or whether the friend is at home. There is no point in wasting precious time and energy on a useless errand. Plenty of time should always be allowed for planned outings, so that no one has to rush for a bus or train – or feel furiously frustrated at having missed it.

In some areas, including Southampton, Grimsby, Bolton, Coventry and Gosport, free or reduced fare travel facilities on public transport are known to be available for the blind, the disabled and the elderly, so it may be worth checking with the local welfare authorities for similar concessions in other districts too. But for many disabled people the chance of getting out and about requires more than extra time and thought.

Much knowledge and experience of the problems which affect the physically disabled when they want to get out and about has been collected by the Joint Committee on Mobility for the Disabled, which was formed by over twenty organizations in 1961. This Committee concerns itself not only with transport for the physically disabled, both as drivers and as passengers, with wheelchairs, training of disabled drivers, and the extra expenses of running their own vehicles for people to whom these are not a luxury but a necessity, but also with the uncaring attitude of the general public, and the ignorance of architects in designing buildings with suitable access for the disabled, and the equally disturbing ignorance of at least some physically disabled people about concessions and helpful arrangements (like exemption from rating charges for garages and ground-floor bathrooms and other house alterations, etc.). Their leaflet *Travel for the Severely Disabled* contains much useful information based on experience and lists special devices, including ways to enter a vehicle from a wheelchair (sliding or turning seats); lifts or hoists to transfer a disabled person from his wheelchair into a car; or even ramps and heightened roofs which enable a wheelchair-bound passenger to get into a car. Up-to-date information about actual equipment of this sort can be obtained from the NHS Rehabilitation Centre or Consultant through the disabled person's own GP, from *Equipment for the Disabled* (see page 21), or from the Information Officer, Information Service for the Disabled, Vincent House, Vincent Square, London, SW1.

Vehicles for disabled drivers

The most convenient and adaptable form of personal transport for anyone in any but the most extreme traffic jams is a motor-car. A physically disabled driver with a Government-issued vehicle may find himself exempt from road fund tax and certain other ordinary driving expenses, but his car will be a vital and still rather expensive item of essential equipment if he wants to be independent.

It is thought that there are between 35,000 and 50,000 disabled drivers in the UK. Approximately 6,000 of them use the motor-cars and nearly 20,000 the 'tricycles' issued to them by the Department of Health and Social Security on the recommendation of a hospital consultant because they have lost the use of their legs or have other disabilities which might preclude them from going to work if they have no transport of their own.

Disabled drivers are not restricted to the use of the Government-sponsored tricycles and cars (which are mainly made available to war pensioners or where more than one person in the family is entitled to official aid with personal transport). If they opt out of the scheme, the Department of Health and Social Security will pay for the conversion of any motor-car to hand controls, contributing up to £90 for this purpose. The Disabled Drivers Association will advise on suitable conversions. Two of the best-known firms in this field are Reselco Invalid Carriages Ltd (262 King Street, London, W6) whose directors are themselves polio victims and therefore know the problems involved only too well from personal experience, and Feeny & Johnson (Wembley, Middlesex). But garages in all parts of the country may be able to submit plans for acceptable conversions of standard cars to hand controls.

Driving a motor-car in modern road conditions can be a tricky matter for anybody, but a survey carried out by the Consumers' Association found that the adaptations for the physically disabled add an extra dimension of discomfort, inconvenience and loneliness. Even then, however, any vehicle (tricycle or motor-car) is still preferable to doing without private transport altogether.

Disabled drivers who already hold a driving licence and can continue to drive their own car or have it – or a new one – adapted may have to take a new driving test. New drivers must take a driving test like anyone else but must inform the Ministry of Transport of their disability when they apply. Special lessons on adapted cars are available from the British School of Motoring at their training centre for the disabled (269 Kensington High Street, London, W8) and at least one such car is said to be at the disposal of each of their centres throughout the country on request.

An organization with special experience in this field is the Disabled Drivers Association (Ashwellthorpe Hall, Ashwellthorpe, Norwich). Membership of any of its ninety-eight local branches costs 15s 0d. per annum and confers access to this clearing house for many of the problems which beset disabled drivers, including information about hotels and parking facilities and a platform from which to air complaints.

Another useful source of information is the AA *Hotel Guide for the Disabled* (free to members of the Automobile Association). It lists hotels, guesthouses and restaurants, and gives helpful advice on parking concessions, breakdown services and Ministry-approved repairers of cars for the disabled.

Existing concessions for disabled drivers mean that they are exempt from road fund tax, can get special parking concessions from their local welfare authorities by means of a special car badge and can take their vehicles to the Continent free of charge. Those with Ministry-issued cars and tricycles get free insurance and maintenance as well as a small contribution towards running costs.

Transport for non-drivers

For many of the physically disabled, driving their own car is an impossible dream. They may be too young or, as they grow up, too unwieldy to climb into a car. They may be too old or too much disabled or have lost the use of a hand.

For them, personal mobility must depend on what help they can get from other people: not only the lift offered by a neighbour or a friend, or the voluntary car pool often run by the ladies of a voluntary society, the social club, or Church, or, more often, the ambulance from hospital to take them for treatment.

These disabled passengers often cannot travel without their

wheelchairs and therefore can only be driven in cars or vans which have been specially adapted for them. An electric hoist like the Burvill (£85 from S. Burvill & Son, see Appendix for address) will lift or lower the heaviest person slowly into or out of a car and can be permanently mounted on the roof.

One helpful organization which was originally founded to mobilize a team of volunteer car drivers and motor-cycle riders to help in cases of medical emergencies is the Volunteer Emergency Service (52 Mollison Drive, Wallington, Surrey; see Appendix for telephone number).

Now its services have expanded into the more social sphere of providing transport for outings and even for holidays for physically disabled people, sometimes at the behest of one of the London boroughs, sometimes following private requests. Some of their drivers have been specially trained to take responauts and other severely handicapped people for outings. These include theatres, race meetings, holidays, even a river trip. Other drivers, many of them housewives, specialize in driving spastics on outings as well as to monthly club meetings. Although London-based, drivers from the VES have driven patients for 450-mile trips when asked. But their main sphere of activity is within driving distance of their homes.

Other providers of transport for the disabled are many of the local branches of the Women's Royal Voluntary Service. The WRVS network extends all over the country, and letters and requests from individuals are welcomed, especially if they make known a genuine need for help. Many physically disabled people may already know their local WRVS members who may have visited them in the course of providing meals-on-wheels, visiting them at home, arranging outings, or bringing out-work to house-bound invalids.

The Rotary Clubs, too, often provide transport for the disabled, and say that trips to the country, transport to hospital, to clubs or classes or to visit friends and relations are most in demand, although they have, for instance, also taken a boy to see a professional football match. They also often help with special shopping expeditions, often out of normal hours, for the disabled. Local welfare officers are usually aware of what facilities are available from this source.

Access to public buildings, shops, etc.

Getting there is, however, not the whole story. It's never enough just to travel hopefully. What happens to the physically disabled when they arrive?

One answer, straight from personal experience, is given in a book called *London for the Disabled*, by Freda Bruce Lockhart, published by Ward Lock & Co. at 6s. 9d., and obtainable from the Central Council for the Disabled.

The author is writing about what she knows only too well, and gives helpful advice and information not only for Londoners but for people in all parts of the country. She mentions the need to plan outings, to discover whether people in wheelchairs can negotiate entrances and staircases as well as lavatories in shops, theatres, and other public places, to arrange for permission to use the goods lifts if available or the luggage lift (by prior arrangement with the Station Master) in railway stations. Even long-distance travel is possible with careful prior planning: in the goods van of a train, for instance, or by special arrangement with an airline.

Nor is London the only town to be documented in this way. Similar booklets have been prepared for Norwich, Cambridge, and Birmingham. Now, under a project called 'Access for the Disabled', the Central Council for the Disabled (34 Eccleston Square, London, SW1.) is preparing guides for other towns. So far, Coventry, York, Hastings and St Leonards, Oxford, Bath, Birmingham, Cambridge, Norwich, Exeter, Leeds, Manchester, Dublin, and Aberdeen have already joined the list which will eventually cover seventy towns and cities in the UK.

Shopping in crowded stores can present very special difficulties to the physically disabled. But Sainsbury's, for instance, have made some suggestions to help these potential customers. Naturally, they advise them to shop at quiet periods, and offer to provide help for people in wheelchairs at such times, if they wish to select commodities for themselves. Early mornings or when no one else thinks of shopping are usually best. At busy periods, they suggest that arrangements are made through the manager for a member of the staff to assemble the disabled shopper's goods and arrange for payment at the check-out point, and they will take the load out to a vehicle if it is parked near by.

Other shops may well offer similar opportunities if they are approached in time and given a chance to help. The Army & Navy Stores, for instance, even provide wheelchairs for disabled shoppers and specialize in suitable goods (see page 41).

Before Christmas and at certain other times of the year, many shops (including branches of Boots, Woolworths and some department stores) have a special shopping evening when disabled people can shop in organized groups, away from the bustle of the crowds. These excursions are usually under the auspices of a local club for the disabled which means that transport is also provided.

For the blind

Guide dogs

The whole problem of mobility for the blind is not so much, as with the people mentioned above, one of movement as one of direction.

The title of 'man's best friend' is probably more deserved by a well-trained guide dog for the blind than by any over-pampered lap-dog or fashionable breed of the moment. The only trouble is that there are never quite enough to go round.

There are approximately 700 guide dogs in the UK at any one time and usually up to 300 people waiting for them. The working life of one such dog is only about nine years which means much heartbreak when one faithful companion dies, especially if he can't be replaced for a while.

Training a guide dog is an expert business, estimated to cost something like £250 each time. Each dog is eventually paired to its future owner at one of three residential centres of the Guide Dogs for the Blind Association (83-89 Uxbridge Road, Ealing, London, W5). But they are chiefly of use to blind people who are otherwise fit and well and able to control a dog. Their upkeep can cost up to £1 per week.

Long cane

Until September 1969 only a few hundred blind people had received training in orientation and mobility based on the use of the long-cane technique; training in the use of these rigid canes is essential. Since then the setting up by the Royal National

Institute for the Blind in association with St Dunstan's and the Birmingham Royal Institute for the Blind of a National Mobility Centre in Birmingham means that more instructors will be available to local welfare authorities and schools for the blind.

What the blind long-cane user has to learn is not only how to wield the cane rhythmically as he walks, swinging it from side to side so as to extend his awareness of his surroundings by a whole stride as he moves, but also to avoid hurting other people as he does so. With experience, he should be able to pick up information from his cane's lightest touch.

Ultrasonic devices

During the last few years, some blind people with good hearing have been carefully taught to increase their mobility by using a hand-held ultrasonic torch which (rather like the electronic devices described on page 109) emits sounds to register what the bearer cannot see within a radius of up to 20ft. It costs £70, but requires almost a new sixth sense to disentangle and interpret its sound patterns.

Chapter 5

Work

To some people work may continue to mean boring or unpleasant tasks in order to earn an essential living. Why work at all, when the welfare state provides what is virtually a guaranteed minimum income for the unemployed and the unemployable in the shape of unemployment pay, sickness or supplementary benefit – provided, that is, that they are of the privileged sex (male – with an occasional allowance for the unmarried female) and the privileged age group (under sixty-five)?

But for most of the physically handicapped, as for many other relatively low-paid workers, the income they carry home at the end of the week or the month is only part of the satisfaction they get from working. The contact with other people, the feeling of personal involvement and usefulness to the community, the pride of earning money instead of merely needing it to spend, bring emotional and social satisfactions beyond those of able-bodied people who take their capacity to work for granted.

It is no coincidence that Mary Greaves, a polio victim in early childhood, and housebound for the first part of her adult working life, chose as the theme for her MA thesis 'Satisfactions at Work', and that her recently published book *Work and Disability* explores the subject in depth and pinpoints some of the shortcomings, in particular as they affect the potential manager or professional worker.

There is no common denominator by which certain jobs or professions can be designated as being more suitable for the physically handicapped than others. As a human being, can anyone ever be assumed to be just the sum of his physical abilities or disabilities? Certainly, as a worker, he can only be assessed to the top of his ability or potential, minus his inescapable handicaps. (Occasionally, as in the case of totally deaf people doing noisy jobs, like riveting, calculating machine operating, card punching and copy typing, physical handicap can even be a positive advantage at work.)

Choosing a suitable job must depend at least in part on the age at which the physically disabled person is faced with it. But natural talents and inclinations, educational attainments or potential, and the candidate's physical and domestic situation are important factors to be considered too.

To a school-leaver, the process will be similar to that undergone by his contemporaries. He will need, and get, assistance and advice from his teachers who know him from personal experience. The Youth Employment Officer too will be able to help him.

But the long-distance lorry driver who can no longer carry on with his job because of an accident or illness will generally need assessment and re-training (although it was nice to hear of at least one whose skill and experience were of professional value to the Consumers' Association in their comparative tests on invalid tricycles). A labourer on a building site or a window-cleaner may not have acquired any working skill he can use if he is physically disabled. He will have to be re-trained, as quickly as possible, to do some other job. Work is habit-forming as well as therapeutic: a newly-disabled person can become demoralized almost beyond hope of resuscitation if he is allowed to remain in unproductive idleness for too long.

A man or woman whose professional equipment is brain, knowledge and experience rather than brawn, muscular skill and freedom of movement is likely to be able to continue to work as a doctor, computer operator or teacher provided he can make certain arrangements to side-step the effects of his physical handicap – such as an inability to climb the stairs, umpire cricket matches, visit his patients in their homes or his clients in their offices. Such disabilities are by no means always negligible: they may mean loss of seniority, or career prospects. Comparisons are too invidious and bitter to investigate individually, but they could as fairly be made with the state of not working at all as with the state of affairs before the onset of the physical handicap.

Finding work, training or re-training for a job is not something which should be left to chance for anyone physically disabled. A great many helpful organizations exist, with titles familiar to the point of abbreviation to the initiated. But ignorance of what DRO (Disablement Resettlement Officer), IRU (Industrial Resettlement Unit) or HPR (Handicapped Persons' Register) stand for need not disbar anyone from using them for their own advantage.

Handicapped Persons' Register

This is not a complete list of all the disabled people of working age in the country, even supposing that anyone could agree on a suitable definition of disablement.

The register applies only to disabled persons seeking work. Registration is voluntary but is principally of interest to disabled people hoping to be employed by a firm under the statutory regulation which requires three per cent of the work force to be recruited from the disabled.

Undoubtedly, many physically handicapped people in employment are NOT on the HPR. And, unfortunately, a disproportionately large number of people on the register (nearly ten per cent) are unemployed. But although registration, therefore, cannot be said to guarantee a job, it costs nothing, and may do some good in procuring some knowledge of the local labour market, including the actual finding of employment.

Disablement Resettlement Officer

There are over 1,100 Disablement Resettlement Officers working in employment exchanges in all parts of the country. As their name suggests, they have been trained in the placing of disabled persons in work. The blind have their own Blind Resettlement Officers, trained to take care of their special career problems.

DROs have a two-way responsibility: partly to the physically handicapped for whom they find work (or try to find work) and partly to keep in touch with employers and find suitable staff for them. But their responsibility to the disabled goes beyond finding suitable work. They can also advise them on mechanical aids which can be provided to help a disabled person at work, or to get to work, on facilities for industrial rehabilitation and vocational training if necessary or, if all else fails, on the finding of sheltered employment.

The DRO is not himself a social worker, but he often works

as part of a team which may include a social worker as well as a doctor, psychiatrist or psychologist, and other specialists. Nor need he confine his activities to disabled people on the HPR. His concern is with all the disabled.

Industrial Resettlement Units

The Department of Employment runs a total of twenty-five Industrial Resettlement Units, dealing mainly with training for manual labour and clerical work. There are special schemes for the blind and for the cerebrally palsied (in conjunction with the Spastics Society) and one for handicapped school leavers. But the IRUs do not set out to provide industrial training for work (although this may be incidental to the course). They provide a basis for assessment on which a physically handicapped person can be trained for employment, and if so, what sort of job he is likely to be able to do.

Most courses at IRUs run for six to eight weeks but they can take longer, and are specially planned for each student with a view to helping him resume the habit of work which he may have lost as a result of illness or injury. They are usually a preliminary to attendance at a government training centre or residential centre.

Careers advice and assessment for work

Like any other worker in the free labour market, physically handicapped people find it easier to get jobs if they have some special training or skill which they are able to exercise alongside able-bodied colleagues. Best of all are the scarce skills for which demand remains practically insatiable: even severely disabled university graduates with specialized qualifications in maths and science subjects seem to find jobs and can even sometimes pick and choose among several situations offered.

All careers advice must take into consideration not only the natural talents, inclinations and abilities of the candidates concerned but the state of the labour market. Disappointments and setbacks in finding work are hard on anyone, but especially hard on young people on the threshold of the big world who have yet to establish themselves as responsible adults in their own eyes and those of their parents and teachers. Young, physically-handicapped people often have already to put up with so much frustration in personal independence that a career problem may well seem like the last straw which would break the heart and spirit of even a well-adjusted young man or woman.

It is important to get good careers advice in plenty of time. Teachers at special schools for physically handicapped children should be consulted as early as possible during the pupil's secondary schooling. The old idea of crafts and charity for the physically handicapped is fast dying out, but adequate training for modern skills is imperative if they are to be properly competitive. In most areas, Youth Employment Officers will advise and place young physically handicapped people or have them placed in work by the local employment exchange, sometimes using the Disablement Resettlement Officer as an intermediary.

Probably the most concentrated body of experience on finding suitable work for the disabled has been built up by the Spastics Society, whose Social Work and Employment Department (see Appendix for address) provides a wide variety of services for children, school leavers and adults. These include specialized assessment for spastic children covering the child's all-round physical, psychological, social and educational potential. Children are usually referred there by the local authority which then pays 10gns for the service, but voluntary organizations and parents can ask for the assessments direct.

Vocational and occupational assessment services are also available for teenage and older spastic people. These usually take the form of a short residential course lasting for five or six days. (Local authorities are charged a fee of up to 20gns for the full course.) A careful evaluation is built up for each participant, and a recommendation is made about the likely future level of work in open or sheltered employment, or in a work centre.

Training facilities

Schooling for physically handicapped children has already been discussed in Chapter 3.

Pupils who have been able to attend normal schools successfully should have little difficulty in continuing their professional training alongside their able-bodied contemporaries. They are already experienced adapters.

But special arrangements may have to be made if the school leaver's further training involves leaving home, as in the case of those who intend to go to universities. Belfast, York, Birmingham and Reading Universities are among those which have made special provision for physically disabled students. Brunel has even integrated students in wheelchairs into sandwich courses in mechanical engineering, mathematics and physics. The Disablement Resettlement Officer will often be able to help a would-be student at a commercial or technical college find suitable accommodation.

There are over forty Government training centres to which physically handicapped (as well as the able-bodied) people can go in order to acquire a marketable skill. The courses run for six months or over and prepare their students to take skilled jobs in a large variety of trades ranging over the building and contracting industries to engineering, the motor trade, cabinet-making, men's hairdressing, and many others. One course on light engineering is reserved for the blind. In addition, there are special training courses run by the voluntary organizations themselves, which are subsidized by the Department of Employment: for instance the School of Physiotherapy or the commercial courses run by the RNIB or the basic training programmes in clerical work, engineering etc., run by the Spastics Society at their residential centres in Welwyn and Lancaster.

The bedbound, whether at home, in hospitals or sanatoria, can be helped to train towards employment by the British Council for the Rehabilitation of the Disabled (Tavistock House South, Tavistock Square, London, WC1). The Council deals with up to 2,000 people each year – of whom nearly three-quarters eventually become self-supporting – often arranging courses of study through correspondence colleges or even by personal tuition. Their services are free to the student and are paid through the local authority in whose area he resides. Some of their success stories include a civil servant who became a teacher, a driver who became a quantity surveyor, a welder who became a book-keeper, but their work spreads across more than a hundred categories of jobs (many in open employment) to suit people of all kinds of backgrounds who have become disabled by accident or illness.

Sheltered employment

In many – but not all – parts of the country, the physically handicapped person who wants to work may be able to find a job in sheltered employment through the DRO or some other social agency. There, he can earn wages varying from modest to average, with the possibility of fitting himself eventually for similar work in open employment.

Probably Remploy is the best known of the employers of the physically handicapped in sheltered workshops, but they are only one – although the largest – of a number of firms providing services for industry in this way.

The work done may be one of a range of tasks considered physically appropriate to the workers and useful to industry, from furniture-making to tool-making, drilling, inspection of components, and other engineering tasks.

For those physically handicapped people who find even sheltered employment beyond them, many local authories run smaller (diversionary) work centres. Here, too, the work is usually subcontracted to industry, and may include packaging, sorting, or craft work. Wages are at pocket-money level (£1 10s. 0d. to £1 19s. 11d.) so that the physically handicapped worker still qualifies for his full social security payment but finds, with free meals and transport, that it compares quite favourably with other sheltered employment.

Work at home

Even gluing plastic toys, sewing at piece-work rates or threading beads, may seem better to the totally housebound than sitting idle all day, especially if it brings in more than a little pocket-money. Generally speaking, however, working for money at home is not to be recommended except for people with the most exceptional talents or circumstances.

Private initiative is often rewarded but, as has already been pointed out by many people, the housebound disabled may find themselves in competition with housebound mothers of small children and other homeworkers.

One firm which sells toys, baby clothes, handbags, gloves, baskets, woodwork, tablemats, pottery, and so on, made by disabled people is the Homebound Craftsmen's Shop (25a,

Holland Street, London, W8). If you can make something which might fit in, send a sample to Miss Jean Harvey, herself a polio victim. She'll buy anything she considers suitable, at trade terms, and may well keep you in regular business after that. Now that similar craft shops – not necessarily specializing in things made by the disabled – are thriving in towns all over the UK you might also try to show your own home-made cushions, toys, leather goods or whatever to the proprietor there, to see whether you can land yourself with a steady sales outlet locally.

Chapter 6

Leisure and holidays

Planning what to do in one's spare time sounds like a dream for busy people with plenty of hobbies and interests, but the reality is often too much like the indiscriminate spending of a fortune suddenly acquired on the football pools. Without a great deal of thought and planning there may not be much to show for it in the end and nothing much to be proud of either.

It's important to look at the problem realistically. During most people's working life, time is at a premium. To be able to spend unlimited time on a stamp collection or photography, golf or cooking, visiting friends or writing a book may sound like an unattainable paradise.

But time is not the only factor to consider in choosing hobbies for the physically handicapped or the housebound elderly.

Their health and physical condition is obviously important. Can they get out of the house fairly easily? Even if their established pursuits like tennis or travelling have become impossible, could they not now serve as a spring-board for a new interest? It may not sound so exciting to play golf as rugger, to take part in a correspondence magazine as to meet new people in the flesh, to listen to records as to go to concerts, to garden in a raised window-box as to collect rare Alpine plants, but all such hobbies can become new starting points.

Cost is important too. Money may be less plentiful now than it was, especially if physical handicap has meant unavoidable expenditure on transport or household and nursing help, using up cash previously set aside for antique buying, dog breeding or butterfly collecting. The regular salary or wage packet may have been superseded by a less ample pension or social-security payment.

There are many difficulties in the way of leisure-time activities for the physically disabled but many of them can be overcome, provided he or she is willing to be adaptable. Probably the most difficult cases are those people whose work or sport was frankly their main interest in life and who are now cut off by their developing illness or condition from the only thing they ever considered worth doing.

It may seem appallingly difficult to arouse a new interest in someone who is homebound or even unable to leave his bed but it's well worth trying out quite a number of subjects, rather like making a first garden in the kind of wrecked builder's yard usually found surrounding a new house one has just moved into. Somewhere, underneath all that unpromising rubble, there'll be soil in which plants may grow eventually. But it'll take much trial and error, patient effort and many setbacks before the most suitable ones are discovered.

Interests and pastimes for the housebound

Embroidery, painting, chess, card games, knitting are all worth trying. The British Red Cross Society's two booklets, *Aids for the Disabled* (which can be ordered direct from them at Grosvenor Crescent, London, SW1) and *Home-made Aids for the Disabled* suggest a number of occupational aids to help invalids who may not be able to hold embroidery or sewing, cards or a needle for threading.

Making things is satisfying in itself, whether the results are modern collages or salt sculpture or traditional items like pincushions, padded clothes hangers or raffia baskets. For the tidy-minded, there's model-making or tapestry, with something impressive to show at the end for all that expenditure of cash and endeavour.

Reading is such a top favourite with many homebound people that care must be taken not to overload them with books, newspapers and magazines. As with food and sleep, enough is as good as a feast, and too much is self-defeating. Local libraries operate a house-bound readers' service which delivers and collects up to six books at a time, keeping a special record of the invalid's interests. Application forms for this service are available from the librarians.

Books are more enjoyable if they've been picked to interest the reader, especially if he reads slowly, and wants to get the utmost enjoyment or benefit from his reading. Librarians are usually very co-operative and knowledgeable. Book reviews are a useful guide to what's new and what other people are reading and thinking about (if not necessarily to what's best).

People with failing eyesight will be able to get the Ulverscroft Large Print Books (21s. 0d. per volume from F. A. Thorpe (Publishing) Ltd, Station Road, Glenfield, Leicester). Their type faces are about twice as large as ordinary print. Their list includes mysteries, romances, Westerns, fiction as well as non-fiction, and some books for children between eleven and fifteen, but most of their books are popular rather than adventurous or highbrow. A large-print hymn book is also available.

Book-stands can be bought or made from instructions from one of the two Red Cross booklets already mentioned. Simple page-turners can be activated by a headband, or hand-held to scrape the page over. Some automatic page-turners ranging in price from £7 to over £100 were tested by the Research Institute for Consumer Affairs, and although they concluded that no ideal page-turner really exists the results of their findings have been included in the *Equipment for the Disabled* (see page 21) published by the National Fund for Research into Crippling Diseases. Certainly, few things can be more irritating than a page-turner which doesn't function or which turns over more than one page at a time, just as one has settled in for a good read.

A predilection for TV-viewing would seem to be a good pastime for the physically disabled, shared as it is by most able-bodied people. But the radio must not be forgotten nor thought of as only a provider of background noise. A browse through the *Radio Times* will reveal a choice of all sorts of goodies, not only plays and interesting talks but stimulating discussions and the opportunity to learn a new language or swot for 'O' and 'A' levels. The BBC is particularly conscious of the special appeal it has for the homebound and disabled. One other useful service it provides is a monthly newsletter of play précis and of the Sunday serial, so that deaf viewers too can follow TV plays even if they can't hear some, or all, the dialogue.

A new hobby or interest may well be fanned and nourished by one of the numerous specialist magazines. Not all of them are to be found on every bookstall but they can usually be ordered if asked for. If you're not sure whether teaching or pop music, beekeeping or filming, archaeology or china-collecting, drama or architecture is catered for, you may well find the answer in *Willing's Press Guide*. It's pricey at £3. 3s. 0d., but available at most public libraries and lists many more publications than you'll ever have dreamed of, or have time to read.

Local newspapers are funds of information about issues, trends and events near by, and local societies previously never even heard of may well be worth joining. They include consumer groups, political associations, debating societies, camera clubs, study groups researching into the history of the district. A letter to the editor can often air a grievance, and maybe even help to remedy it – which gives a most satisfactory feeling of involvement and usefulness.

Even for the totally bedbound, life can be made more interesting by arranging for regular visiting. Conversation can sometimes be sticky, so it's a good idea to have one or two conversational standbys (not the weather) in the shape of something topical to discuss: an item from the news, or something you've read or what your visitor is doing in the school, the job, the home he has outside your four bedroom walls. A bird-table placed where the invalid can see it can be engrossing, and less demanding than an individual pet.

A bi-monthly magazine run by and for the housebound and physically handicapped is *The Road*. It is available from the editor, Miss Peggy Harding, 64 Berkeley Road, Fishponds, Bristol, at 5s. 6d. for a year's subscription, and may be another way of resuming contact with the big world outside, including the chance of acquiring a pen-friend, or doing some bedside shopping.

The blind

Since the days of Homer, blindness has been no bar to the exercise of natural talent. A blind artist recently described the paintings he makes of scenes he remembers from the time when he could see. He makes deep indentations in his paper with a hard pencil, then fills these in from a palette of twenty-four colours prepared for him by his wife. A blind folk singer recently visited the USA with his specialized repertoire of Western-type songs. There are many examples of blind writers who have dictated or typed their works for other people to read. The blind are not physically disabled in the way that the term applies to other people. They can do things, provided they know how. Probably their best source of advice and help will come from the local authority's home teachers, as well as from the Royal National Institute for the Blind.

All blind people can get a free radio under the British Wireless Fund for the Blind, and free licences. They can also get the *Radio Times* in braille, books and magazines transposed into braille, and talking books.

The RNIB's Sales Department has a catalogue and price list, *Apparatus and Games*, containing some 300 aids and items which have either been specially made or adapted for the blind. They include card games, dominoes, chess, solitaire, bézique, etc, all at fairly low prices as blind people can buy them at a third of cost price. Two electronic devices, the Sound Beacon (£1) or the Light Probe (£1 19s. 0d.) emit sound to register what sighted people can see (see Fig. 12). The Sound Beacon can be used as a direction and object finder, for instance to locate a lawn-mower in the garden; the Light Probe can tell you whether electric appliances like radios, tape-recorders, etc. are switched on, whether the baby's bottle is full, half-full or nearly empty, whether there's writing on a page.

With 12,000 people in the UK losing their sight each year, the RNIB's services may not always be known to all the people who could make use of them.

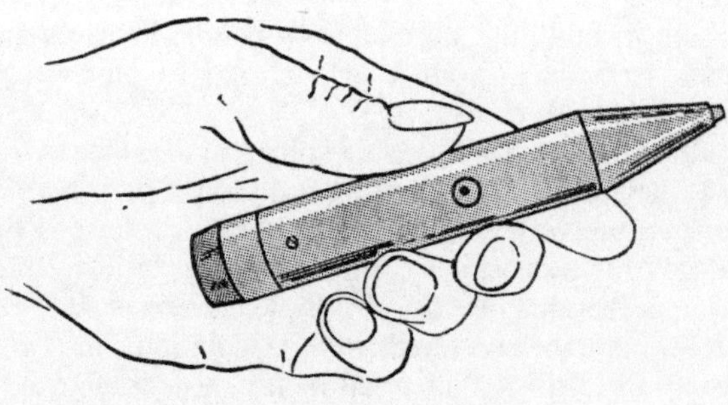

Fig. 12 A light probe. A photo-electric cell which converts light into varying sound frequencies so that blind people can measure light.

Organized leisure activities

You may never have heard of many of these until you need them, but there are many ingenious solutions to the problem of organizing a whole range of activities for the physically disabled, both at home and outside their home.

An impressive list which includes music, gardening, listening to the radio, record-playing, printing, pony riding, swimming, golf, a world-wide pen club for multiple sclerosis patients, and a tape club as well as a number of local sports clubs in many parts of the country is available from the Information Service for the Disabled, Vincent House, Vincent Square, London, SW1. It also lists a number of useful books for physically handicapped people who are interested in gardening. Growing things is a favourite occupation with many elderly or physically disabled people, and need not mean ownership of an extensive garden. Even bending and stooping can be virtually eliminated with clever planning, elevated, built-up flower beds and window boxes. Special aids can be bought from the Army & Navy Stores mail-order catalogue for the physically disabled. A permanent demonstration garden for elderly or disabled people can be seen at Syon Park, Middlesex.

Clubs and societies

It has already been pointed out that a physically disabled person has not suddenly opted out of the human race when it comes to those interests and hobbies which are common ground: political, social, professional, and so on. The only special factor to bear in mind is how he or she will get to the meetings, and whether they are held in buildings accessible to people in wheelchairs or on crutches, with or without a helper, and to plan or ask for appropriate help with transport.

What all sufferers from certain physical handicaps have in common is their difficulty in getting around on their own. Often, their lives become very confined. This state of affairs is to some extent catered for by social meetings arranged by local branches of such organizations as the Multiple Sclerosis Society, the British Rheumatism and Arthritis Association, in swimming galas held by the British Polio Fellowship, and similar activities, social, therapeutic or just plain neighbourly (see Appendix for addresses).

As so often, Londoners seem to be particularly well provided for with clubs – though in this case the area involved stretches from Havering in Essex to Kingston, Surrey, and from Barnet, Herts, to Bromley in Kent. The Greater London Association for the Disabled (183 Queensway, London, W2) has compiled a list of over 500 local social clubs for the disabled, the deaf, dumb or blind. It mentions meeting-places, dates, and whom to contact for details of transport facilities. The total cost of the complete list is £2 2s. 0d., but individual borough sections cost only 5s. 0d. each, and the whole work is to be revised annually.

Clubs for the physically disabled often have a function which goes beyond the purely social one by playing a therapeutic role in aiding adaption to normal life in the community, and the PHAB Clubs (see page 82) for young people up to twenty-five provide a chance for contact between the physically handicapped and able-bodied.

It was because the disabled tend to lead sheltered lives that the Spastics Society's '62 Clubs were started. These are run by the cerebrally palsied themselves, and often provide them with their first-ever opportunity of making decisions, arranging club programmes and outings, laying on transport, and coping with their own finances. Many thrive on this sort of practical experience: acquire a new spurt of self-confidence, learn to speak in public, handle other people singly and in groups, and benefit personally from this new extension of themselves. There are now over thirty active local branches of the '62 Clubs – over 1,500 members – with membership rates generally between 10s. and 15s. per annum. For addresses of local clubs, and other details, write to William Hargreaves, Clubs Officer, The Spastics Society, 16 Fitzroy Square, London, WIP 5HQ.

Fund-raising is often the best-publicized of the activities of organizations for the physically handicapped, but it must never be thought of as the only one. Most of the national organizations listed in the Appendix have local branches whose activities may include communal outings, theatre visits and even holidays. Voluntary organizations like Task Force or the Community Volunteer Service welcome help from any quarter: a blind boy was cheerfully set to helping crippled children with their swimming practice, and there is always scope for volunteer knitters, tea-makers, friendly natterers or readers-aloud.

Details of local clubs, societies or voluntary organizations are usually available from local libraries.

Classes

Learning or doing something new is a satisfying occupation for most people, providing them with a fine sense of achievement and, usually, an ever-present desire to do better!

Adult education classes exist in most parts of the country. Often, classes can be laid on specially if a minimum of fifteen people will undertake to attend them regularly. Subjects vary, not merely according to demand (or estimated demand) from students but also depending on the supply of teachers. The specialist on Roman Britain can hardly be expected to teach Spanish if he doesn't know any, nor would it be possible to run a course on Continental cookery in a place where no cooking facilities exist.

There are special classes for the physically handicapped in many areas. They are usually run by the local welfare authorities (rather than the education authority), with transport provided, if asked for, by the welfare department. Again, Inner London leads the field, with more than 580 non-vocational welfare classes in subjects which include pottery, music and movement, needle-craft, wood-work, cookery, clay modelling, gardening (indoors and out), art, old-tyme dancing and current affairs.

Some young disabled people can enjoy the residential week-long courses run by PHAB, the National Association of Youth Clubs. These and other interesting residential courses are listed in six-monthly calendars issued by the National Institute of Adult Education (35 Queen Anne Street, London, W1M OBL) at 2s. 6d. each.

Holidays

Everybody benefits from a holiday and a change of scenery. This applies to the physically handicapped as well as to the person normally looking after the disabled person, especially if he or she is a loving and dutiful relative who may not have thought himself or herself entitled to any respite. In most areas local authorities will provide temporary accommodation for a severely handicapped person, often through a voluntary agency, in a hospital, holiday home, nursing home or similar place.

But many physically handicapped people are quite capable of enjoying a holiday away from home. Even severely handicapped people (including at least one respiratory polio case who normally lives in an iron lung) can go on holiday with their families, provided everything is carefully planned to their physical limitations. Obviously, problems of access, ground-floor bedrooms or large lifts, WCs and bathrooms must be within the disabled person's competence.

A great deal depends on the extent of disablement, the general state of health and spirits, the independence of the disabled person, and whether he or she is travelling alone or with a helper. Ted Appleton, polio-afflicted travel agent, is adventurous enough to travel on the Continent, but suggests that air travel is best and that resorts should be chosen with care for their accessibility to the nearest airport.

The airline company must be told in advance if a passenger is physically disabled, and preferably should be reminded again a week before the actual journey to ensure that he is properly received by the ground staff and wheeled aboard the aircraft before the other passengers. Wheelchairs should be as light as possible as they count as part of the precious luggage allowance (44 lbs on a tourist flight).

Sea cruising is another recommended way of travelling, but the shipping company must be informed of the extent of the passenger's disability. Companies usually refuse responsibility for any accident which may ensue as a result, but that omniscient Information Officer of the DLF will provide details of where to apply for cover for individual cases. Incidentally, a large liner usually carries a doctor and medical staff which could be useful though – one hopes! – not vital to the success of the holiday.

Some travel agencies arrange special package holidays for the physically disabled. The Erna Low Travel Service Ltd (47 Old Brompton Road, London, SW7) have some experience in this field and will tailor a holiday specifically for a physically handicapped person.

Some good suggestions for holidays for the elderly, including some for the disabled, used to be published by the BBC's *Home This Afternoon* programme, a sad loss to many housebound people. Occasionally, *Woman's Hour* may be able to fill this gap in the future.

Probably the most useful detailed source of addresses for holidays for the disabled in the UK is a little book *Holidays for the Physically Handicapped,* published jointly by the Central Council for the Disabled and the British Red Cross Society. It costs 3s. 6d. from either of its sponsors. Holidays are grouped to show how they might suit people with varying degrees of physical handicap under the following headings: Specially designed accommodation, No help available (which means bringing your own if you need it), Limited personal help, Number of incontinents accepted (in some cases only with accompanying help), Night attention, Nursing care, and Holidays for large parties. Understandingly, since the needs of the physically handicapped are so varied, the book provides names and addresses of voluntary organizations who have compiled their own lists of hotels, boarding houses, nursing homes, camps, and so on. Diabetics, epileptics, severely disabled ex-servicemen and women, heart and stroke cases, or people suffering from multiple sclerosis, muscular dystrophy and spastics can all find accommodation where they are accepted and suitably catered for.

Chapter 7

Money and grants

One of the greatest burdens many physically-disabled people have to bear is the fact that they live in conditions of great hardship and personal poverty, mainly because they are, or have become unemployed. There may be a number of reasons why they have become unemployable: their previous job required strength rather than skill, they are getting too old for many kinds of work, or they cannot cope with the wear and tear of getting to and holding down a full-time job.

In modern society, this seems to be adding insult to injury, especially from the social aspect. The financial rewards of work can be, at least to some extent, made up in social security payments, pensions and insurances, but a job – whether as a truck-driver, a veterinary surgeon, a civil servant or a nurse – acts as a kind of identity card.

Many people not at work – including retired people and house-bound housewives as well as the disabled – feel that they are virtually shut off from the general work- and achievement-orientated community because they are not in paid employment. A very great personal awareness of identity and individuality is often necessary to maintain self-respect and even equilibrium in such circumstances, especially if they are made even harder to bear by shortage of money.

In addition, physical handicap can be expensive. Even on an average weekly household budget, and despite the free medical attention and other help provided either through the local authority, a voluntary society, or a combination of the two, physical handicap may mean a higher-than-average expenditure on food, transport, household or sickroom help, heating, etc. Plus, one might add, a greater need to be cheered by the things money *can* buy – if not full health – freedom from want, a TV set, food for the beloved cat or budgie or the trusty guide dog, cigarettes or stamps, a tape-recorder or an electric blanket, items from a mail-order firm's catalogue without worrying that essential resources will have been irretrievably wasted if the article ordered is unsatisfactory.

Social-security payments

Living in a welfare state may be just a phrase to some people, especially if they are ill-housed, uncomfortable and generally unhappy. Yet it must be remembered that the present state of affairs is an improvement on the stark past when men, women and children could literally starve to death.

Nowadays, every man, woman or child in the UK existing below a certain income is entitled to draw some benefit, allowance or pension from the State under some category or other. Unfortunately, many people do not know what their rights and entitlements are, and some do not choose to exercise them or to explore the possibility of claiming for them under some heading other than the one they first thought of. Often, such people may be too depressed and ill to care. Sometimes, too, they can't be bothered or don't want to expose themselves to the chance of being refused.

It is true that there is not, as yet, one single scale of financial support for everyone who needs it. Scales for sickness and disability benefit, supplementary assistance and old-age pensions are laid down nationally, but it is the local offices of the Department of Health and Social Security who pay them out. Local authorities' welfare departments can also offer financial aid, and many of them interpret the rules on this generously.

But none of the benefits and allowances come automatically. All have to be claimed, either on a form available from local post offices or on application to the welfare departments of the local authority. A disabled father of a family may be able to obtain assistance with the rent or help with mortage repayments or an allowance to buy fuel. Sometimes the local education authority will provide a clothing grant for the children if the family income is below a certain level, as well as free school meals. There are also discretionary allowances, which can be made on recommendation, to buy large items like beds or blankets, or regular weekly payments for special diets or necessary domestic help.

What are the actual money sums paid out to individuals for social-security payments?

The basic amounts vary according to the age and status (married or single, householder or in rented accommodation) of the recipient, and at present (June 1970) range from approximately £2 16s. 0d. for a sixteen- or seventeen-year-old living with his parents or in someone else's household to £7 17s. 0d. for a married couple.

Such sums do not look adequate when they are compared with average national earnings. But they are not strictly comparable. A wage and salary earner must spread his weekly income to maintain his wife and/or other dependants, pay rent, and meet his mortgage or hire-purchase commitments. Only the money which is left over after these fixed expenditures have been covered is his to spend as he wishes. On the other hand, the social-security payment, whether in the shape of pension, unemployment or sickness benefit, supplementary allowance or industrial injury benefit, is tailored to the recipient's individual commitments by additions for dependants, rent, etc.

The social security net is comprehensive and interlocking. Sometimes public attention centres on its abuses. But care is already taken that a man cannot claim unfairly twice over for the same problem, i.e. that he does not get sickness benefit as well as unemployment pay, or that, even if he meets twice with a severe accident, he does not get more than one 100% disability pension.

Often, however, a physically disabled person can be entitled to more than one benefit for the same basic reason. He might, for instance, qualify for a disablement benefit as well as an unemployability supplement. But if he already gets a full allowance for a dependent wife as a war-disabled pensioner, he cannot also claim a full allowance for her if he becomes unemployed.

More poignant than the danger of someone trying to claim illegally or unknowingly two social-security payments where he is only, strictly speaking, entitled to one, is the prospect of a case of hardship slipping through the net altogether, either through ignorance of what can be done to help or through deficiences in the system with all its numerous individual variants. Social workers consider this to be a much more obvious and usual risk, especially since changes in rates, and now the advent of the promised earnings-related insurance scheme as well as the invalidity pension and attendance allowance for the most severely disabled, often mean that only civil servants and professionals may know what the actual day-to-day allowances are.

Leaflets about the benefit schemes and claim forms can be obtained from post offices. The local office of the Department of Health and Social Security should be able to help with advice, and so will the local branches of the voluntary societies (see Appendix for their central addresses). The local office of the Citizens' Advice Bureau too should be able to work out individual entitlements for pensions, benefits and allowances, and explain how they can be claimed.

Benefits and allowances

At the receiving end, a pension (which is the result of weekly contributions having been paid by an employed person towards a State insurance against sickness, unemployment or old age) or an allowance (which the State makes available to people in need) may look much the same. Both come in the shape of money – usually in an order book to be presented at a nominated post office – which must be spent on essential food, clothing, and other necessities of life. Neither will ever seem to be quite large enough for all one's needs, but the intention is to provide a minimum basic living allowance according to a complicated calculation of individual need, irrespective of personal merit or misery.

The actual amounts come under various headings: sickness benefit (paid in full only to anyone who has contributed to the national insurance scheme for a minimum of 156 weeks), retirement pension (paid to men over sixty-five and women over sixty), and industrial injury benefit and disablement benefit (covering all insured workers). All of them can be augmented still further if necessary by unemployability supplement, constant attendance allowance, exceptionally severe disablement allowance, and special hardship allowance, plus allowances to dependent wives and children. Under special circumstances, money for special clothing can also be obtained.

Payments vary according to the origin of the injury or disability for which they are made. A war disablement pension for, say, the loss of a limb will be higher than industrial injury benefit for the same injury. And there is no special benefit whatsoever available to anyone who has suffered the same injury as the result of a traffic accident or illness.

This discrepancy is an understandable cause for grievance and sometimes causes real hardship.

Supplementary benefit can be paid out to young people over the age of sixteen if their total income falls below what is considered the basic minimum. This applies to handicapped sons and daughters who cannot earn money, irrespective of their parents' income.

Benefits and allowances for blind people are somewhat higher than average to meet their above-average essential expenditures. If they are employed they are also entitled to a special personal income tax allowance of £100 p.a.

Disablement income group (DIG)

One of the most glaring gaps in the welfare state is the lack of financial provision for the disabled as people (rather than as ex-servicemen, ex-workers, etc.). This applies particularly to married women with no job outside their homes. An average housewife's work in the home may save her family money which they might have to pay out for domestic help, additional food, clothes and decorating bills if she became disabled. But even then, neither she nor they would qualify for any sort of State aid in respect of her disability.

In the present system, financial support depends on the cause of the disability, for example, whether it is a result of war injury or industrial injury, and not on the disabling effect of the injury or illness. We are faced with the paradox that the increase in medical skill which results in more disabled babies surviving and more accident cases surviving, is accompanied by no financial help for the congenitally disabled or the civilian disabled.

Many of the severely disabled may well prefer to live at home with their own families even though they may be entitled to a free hospital bed under the NHS. This decision can save the State £1000 per annum or even more.

The Disablement Income Group was founded in 1965 to campaign for the rights of all the disabled (physically as well as mentally), for recognition of their special difficulties, and for a national disability income. The group sees this as a matter of common sense as much as compassion: many of the disabled already receive some sort of state aid under one heading or another. A national disability income would be available to all severely disabled people, irrespective of national insurance contributions.

Already, the National Insurance Act 1970 includes a constant attendance allowance for those severely disabled living at home who are unable to do anything for themselves. So DIG is obviously making an impact but it still has a long way to go before its objectives are attained. DIG is not pressing for a pension for invalids, but for people who incur extra costs in their daily lives because of some form of disablement.

For further details write to the Disablement Income Group, Godalming, Surrey. Membership is 2s. 6d. for disabled members and 10s. for non-disabled.

Grants for home improvements

Essential alterations to the home of a physically handicapped person (as outlined in Chapter 2) can be expensive. However, the welfare departments of local authorities are normally equipped to help, and to make cash grants for those alterations which are considered necessary for a physically handicapped person to continue, if he wants, to go on living at home.

Many local authorities will commission their own builders to carry out work, including the widening of doorways, putting in sliding doors, providing a french door to give direct access to a garden, building of ramps, or fixing handles on walls of rooms, stairways and bathrooms. In some cases, private builders can be commissioned to carry out home alterations provided their estimates have been approved by the local welfare department before the work is started.

Financial grants for home improvements can also be made available through many of the voluntary organizations, not necessarily only those concerned with disabilities. Sometimes a professional trust fund or a recognized charity will provide help if approached in the right way.

The British Legion, for instance, with 4,300 local branches will provide financial assistance to ex-servicemen and women and widows of ex-servicemen, disabled or otherwise, in need.

Another helpful organization for home-bound disabled people is Invalids-At-Home (see Appendix for address). Because the organizers believe in helping invalids to remain at home where they can feel more independent and secure, they will provide special grants to cope with emergencies and provide equipment to encourage house-bound invalids to stay in their own environment.

Sheltered housing

One appealing compromise between the difficulty and expense of living on one's own and the dread of becoming dependent and institutionalized in a hostel, home or hospital, can be seen in the sheltered housing schemes now run by some local authorities, and in various stages of planning by certain of the voluntary societies.

Basically, sheltered housing means independence in the shape of one's own flat or bungalow. Yet supervision and emergency care is available if needed. In the case of local authority housing schemes, there are usually some fourteen or so purpose-built living units, mainly inhabited by elderly disabled people, grouped round one warden who visits each tenant once each day, and who can be summoned by means of an emergency bell if needed.

Rents for this kind of accommodation are low, and the schemes are so popular that it cannot by any stretch of imagination be said to be freely or generally available to all who could profit from them. Would-be tenants are nominated by the local authority's welfare department, and should therefore be registered with them.

Several voluntary organizations also now have plans for sheltered housing. Probably the only one to have got off the drawing-board so far is the Heatherly community at Effingham, Sussex, which is being run by the Cheshire Foundation Homes for the Sick (7 Market Mews, London, W1). It is intended to provide housing for younger people (from eighteen to about forty-five or fifty) in these subsidized housing schemes so that one physically handicapped member can live with the rest of his or her able-bodied family, and receive nursing care during the day, if necessary.

Chapter 8

The physically disabled and the community

While I was writing this book I came across very many different stories about individual people with different – or similar – disabilities: stories of personal triumph or desperate and continuing struggle, of professional and domestic success or of bitter financial hardship and deprivation.

But their stories never really added up to point one moral applicable to all. The disabled are every bit as individual as the able-bodied. Sometimes it seemed to me as though everyone in the country were in some way involved with the problems of the disabled. Even Harold Wilson, when premier, mentioned his personal feeling of triumph when a spastic constituent of his at last achieved training and a good job as a computer programmer. Legislation concerning the disabled financially or organizationally is going through Parliament. And the Department of Health and Social Security is conducting a monumental survey into the precise numbers of disabled in the population. Smaller surveys (i.e. Professor Townsend's *The Disabled in Society* or the London borough of Tower Hamlet's *Physical Disability and Community Care*) are widely discussed. Books have been published describing life with a physical handicap (*Stigma, the Experience of Disability*, edited by Paul Hunt, published by Geoffrey Chapman); with multiple sclerosis (*Why Pick On Us?* by Honor Wyatt and George Ellidge, published by Hurst & Blackett); with respiratory polio (*Horizontal Man* by Paul Bates, published by Longmans); as a blind person handicapped as a result of war service (*Blinded in War*, by F. Le Gros Clark, published by the Priory Care and Welfare Library); what it is like to have a cerebrally palsied child (*The Family and the Handicapped Child*, by Sheila Hunt, published by Allen & Unwin); or what it is like to recover from the side effects of a stroke (*Never Say Die*, by Anthony Richards, published by Max Parrish).

On a less personal plane, there have been many publications

from Government departments, voluntary societies, or organizations concerned with specific physical disabilities explaining how to manage. The appointment of a special minister for disablement has even been suggested.

Altogether, there is a great deal of public concern with the subject – understandably so, as this is one problem where individual or group efforts so frequently achieve positive success.

'After all, we live in a welfare state', was the comment most frequently made, sometimes approvingly but mostly bitterly, with the implication that theory and practice are still sometimes far apart. Failures are best blamed on 'them', the anonymous state, the unfriendly government, the faceless (or many-faced?) civil servant. But people who had genuinely benefited from welfare services supplied by the State, whether in the shape of education, professional training, financial support or medical attention, tended to place the credit elsewhere: their parents' or spouse's devotion maybe, or their own initiative, a marvellous doctor, teacher or school, a special aid or gadget, exercises or a miracle cure.

Public awareness

To some extent public awareness of the problems of the physically disabled is already having its effect on matters of general concern. It is beginning to mean that certain – often quite simple – steps are taken to enable physically disabled people to go out and about, to visit public buildings, theatres, museums, shops and WCs, to take jobs (Chapter 5), holidays (Chapter 6), and to enlarge their personal horizons.

It is not always easy. Nor is it possible to state firmly that one kind of disablement may be easier to bear than another: too much depends on whether the disability is congenital or acquired, the age, station in life and profession of the sufferer, his personality, and general background.

The Department of Social Security uses 'loss of faculty' as a yardstick by which to measure the extent of a man's disability, and from that his entitlement to financial support. But administrative convenience is never a good guide to the sufferings of individual people, especially in the present state of the law under which the same disability can attract quite different scales of support according to whether it was contracted at work, on active service, or as the result of a car crash.

For most people it is easier to accept an accident of nature, like the very occurrence of physical disability, than the often haphazard, if not unfair, treatment meted out to it.

For the future

One of the main complaints levied by and on behalf of the physically handicapped is that even where services exist to help them, many people still don't know about them. This may be understandable in the case of a house-bound invalid, but has even been found to affect experienced but busy social workers, doctors, and other professionals, too.

Publications like a local *Directory of Social Services* (see page 19) can be most helpful. On a more general level, so is the Family Welfare Association's annual *Report on the Social Services*. Local libraries should have up-to-date copies of these.

Most encouraging of all are the promised changes in legislation under which local welfare services are eventually to be streamlined into similar shape all over the country, and which promise to provide services and information about them to all who need them, irrespective of whether they have been specifically asked for or not.

The personality factor

But even when a public-spirited, warm-hearted, generous community has done everything that is possible to ensure a tolerable life for its physically-disabled members, one major item stands out: the importance of each individual's own personality.

Like the able-bodied, the physically disabled have many important needs: physical, financial, personal. But the most vital mainspring of all is to have the right disposition and character. A happy nature, and the ability to enjoy one's available capacities and resources for reading or work, social life or an artistic talent, are essential to leading a whole, fulfilled life.

Everyone meets setbacks, and it is often the way these are tackled which reveal and strengthen a person's character. Even partial independence is better than none at all. What parents owe to their disabled children, or the community as a whole to its disabled members, is a safety net to cushion them from disaster in case of failure – not a prison cage. It is only too easy to allow a fatal dependence to develop; it is by no means easy to stand by and allow mistakes to be made, falls taken, time spent trying, trying, and trying again to perform simple actions like dressing, feeding, or looking after oneself because these are the first steps to physical independence.

But in the end the outlook is by no means gloomy. Medical and technological advance have already done much for the physically disabled, but their own, often invincible spirit has gone further and performed near-miracles for some outstanding people among them.

'A physical handicap is much easier to cope with than a personality handicap,' says William Hargreaves, President of the Association of '62 Clubs and Clubs Officer of the Spastics Society. As a spastic himself who has managed to have a successful career and family life, it seems only right to let him have the last word.

Appendix

1 List of organizations and firms mentioned in the text

Abbatt Ltd (Paul & Marjorie) 94 Wimpole Street, London, W1. (for catalogue: PO Box 57, High Wycombe Bucks)	01–580–3884
Access for the Disabled, 34 Eccleston Square, London, SW1	01–834–0747
Aldrex Ltd, Newnham, Glos.	
Army & Navy Stores, 105 Victoria Street, London, SW1.	01–834–1234
Association for Spina Bifida & Hydrocephalus Ltd, 112 City Road, London, EC1.	01–253–2735
Association of '62 Clubs, 16 Fitzroy Square, London, W1 W1P5H9	01–387–9571
British Association of the Hard of Hearing, Hon. Sec. Briarfield, Syke Ings, Iver, Bucks.	01–935–5555
British Council for Rehabilitation of the Disabled, Tavistock House (South), Tavistock Square, London, WC1.	01–387–4037
British Diabetic Association, 3–6 Alfred Place, London, WC1.	01–636–7355
British Epilepsy Association, 3–6 Alfred Place, London, WC1.	01–580–2704
British Legion, 49 Pall Mall, London, SW1.	01–930–8131
British Polio Fellowship, Clifton House, 83/117 Euston Road, London, NW1.	01–387–5851
British Red Cross Society, 14 Grosvenor Crescent, London, SW1.	01–235–5454
British Rheumatism & Arthritis Association, 1 Devonshire Place, London, WIN 2BD	01–935–9905 01–935–9517
British School of Motoring, 269 Kensington High Street, London, W8.	01–937–8272
British Talking Book Service for the Blind, Mount Pleasant, Wembley, Middx.	
British Wireless Fund for the Blind, 224 Gt Portland Street, London, W1.	01–387–5251
Burvill & Son, 143 Hersham Road, Walton-on-Thames, Surrey.	98–27194
Carters, J. & A., 65 Wigmore Street, London, W1.	01–486–3835
Central Council for the Disabled, 34 Eccleston Square, London, SW1.	01–834–0747
Cheshire Foundation Homes for the Sick, 7 Market Mews, London, W1.	01–499–2665
Clos-O-Mat Ltd, 2 Brooklands Road, Sale, Cheshire M33 355.	061–973–6262
Community Service Volunteers, 28 Commercial Street, London, E1.	01–247–8113
Consumers Association, 14 Buckingham Street, London, WC2.	01–930–9921
Cystic Fibrosis Research Trust, Stuart House, 1 Tudor Street, London, EC4.	01–583–0989
Department of Health & Social Security, Alexander Fleming House, London, SE1.	01–407–5522

Disabled Drivers Association, Ashwellthorpe Hall, Ashwellthorpe, Nr Norwich.	0508–41324
Disablement Income Group, Godalming, Surrey.	0486–8–5181
Disabled Living Foundation, Vincent House, Vincent Square, London, SW1.	01–834–8016
Diabetic Association, 3–6 Alfred Place, London, WC1.	01–636–7355
Erna Low Travel Service, 47 Old Brompton Road, London, SW7.	01–589–8881
Family Welfare Association, Denison House, 296 Vauxhall Bridge Road, London, SW1.	01–834–7334
Feeny & Johnson, Wembley, Middx.	
Girl Guides Association, 17 Buckingham Palace Road, London, SW1.	01–834–6242
Goslett & Co., 127 Charing Cross Road, London, WC2.	01–437–7890
Greater London Association for the Disabled, 183 Queensway, London, W2	01–727–4426/7
The Guardian, 192 Gray's Inn Road, London, WC1.	
Guide Dogs for the Blind Association, 83/89 Uxbridge Road, Ealing, London, W5.	01–567–7001
Hammond & Champness Ltd, 159 St John's Street, London, EC1.	01–253–7363
Hobbs & Co, 36 Whitefriars Street, London, EC4.	01–353–1203
Homebound Craftmen's Shop, 25a Holland Street, London, W8.	01–937–3924
Homecraft Supplies Ltd, 27 Trinity Road, London, SW17.	01–672–7070
Hugh Steeper Ltd, Roehampton Lane, London, SW15.	01–788–8165
Information Service for the Disabled, Vincent House, Vincent Square, London, SW1.	01–834–8016
Invalid Children's Aid Association, 126 Buckingham Palace Road, London, SW1.	01–730–9891
Invalids-At-Home, 23 Farm Avenue, London, NW2.	01–452–2074
Jacobs, Young & Westbury, Bridge Road, Haywards Heath, Sussex.	0444–2411
John Bell & Croyden, 50 Wigmore Street, London, W1.	01–935–5555
John Dron, Mountview House, London, N6.	01–340–3211
John Lewis & Co., Oxford Street, London, W1.	01–629–7711
Joint Committee on Mobility for the Disabled, c/o The Spastics Society, 12 Park Crescent, London, W1.	01–636–5020
Kay & Co, Elgar House, Shrubhill Road, Worcester.	0905–26131
Lady Hoare Thalidomide Appeal, 78 Hamilton Terrace, London, NW8.	01–289–0231
Leva Tap Company, 25 Hatton Gardens, London, EC1.	
Medor Ltd, 80 Copenhagen Street, Caledonian Road, London, N1.	01–837–0964
Melaware Ltd, 9 Argyll Street, W1.	01–437–9187
Milan Gowns Ltd, 341 High Road, Wood Green, London, N22.	
Muscular Dystrophy Group, 26 Borough High Street, London, SE1. and Newcastle General Hospital, Westgate Road, Newcastle-upon-Tyne, NE4 6BE.	01–407–5116 0362–38811
Multiple Sclerosis Society, 4 Tachbrook Street, London, SW1.	01–834–8231

National Association for Deaf, Blind and Rubella Children, 61 Senneleys Park Road, Northfield, Birmingham 31
National Association of Youth Clubs, 30 Devonshire Street, London W1. 01–935–2941
National Bureau for Co-operation in Child Care, Adam House, 1 Fitzroy Square, London, W1. 01–387–4263/4/5
National Council of Social Service (Standing Conference of Councils of Social Service) 26 Bedford Square, London, WC1. 01–636–4066
National Deaf Children's Society, 31 Gloucester Place, London, W1H 4EA 01–486–3251/2
National Fund for Research into Crippling Diseases, Vincent House, Vincent Square, London, SW1. 01–834–7001/2
National Institute of Adult Education, 35 Queen Anne Street, London W1M OBL 01–580–3155
National Library for the Blind, 35 Great Smith Street, London, SW1. 01–222–2725 01–799–1782
Noah's Ark Toy Libraries, 21 Gentleman's Row, Enfield, Mddx.
Nylons Unlimited, Gay Street, Bath, Somerset. 0225–60454

P.O.S.M. Project Research, 63 Mandeville Road, Aylesbury, Bucks 0296–81591

Relyon Mattresses, 18 Orchard Street, London, W1. 01–935–0711
Remploy, 415 Edgware Road, London, NW2. 01–452–8020
Research Institute for Consumer Affairs, 20 Buckingham Street, London, WC2. 01–930–3360
Reselco Invalid Carriages Ltd, 262 King Street, London, W6. 01–748–5053
Rotary International in Great Britain & Ireland, Sheen Lane House, Sheen Lane, London, SW14 01–878–0931
Royal National Institute for the Blind, 224 Great Portland Street, London W1. 01–387–5251
Royal National Institute for the Deaf, 105 Gower Street, London, WC1. 01–387–8033
Rubbermaid bathmat, from Carters, J. & A., 65 Wigmore Street, London, W1H OEL 01–486–3835
The Road, Editor, Miss P. Harding, 64 Berkeley Road, Fishponds, Bristol.

St. Dunstan's, PO Box 58, 191 Marylebone Road, London, NW1. 01–723–5021
Scottish Braille Press, Craigmillar Park, Edinburgh 9. 031–667–6230
Selfridges Ltd, Oxford Street, London, W1. 01–629–1234
Scout Association, 25 Buckingham Palace Road, London, SW1. 01–834–6005
Social Work & Employment Department, Spastics Society, Fitzroy Square, London, W1P 5H9. 01–387–9571
Spastics Society, 12 Park Crescent, London, W1. 01–636–5020
16 Fitzroy Square, London, WIP 5HQ. 01–387–9571

Task Force, Clifford House, Edith Villas, London, W14. 01–603–2569
Thalidomide Appeal, 78 Hamilton Terrace, London, NW8 01–289–0231

Ulverscroft Large Print Books, F. A. Thorpe (Publishing) Ltd, Station Road, Glenfield, Leicester. 0533-871552/872828

Volunteer Emergency Service, 52 Mollison Drive, Wallington, Surrey.	01–647–6183
In Emergency only	647–6077
Woman, 185 High Holborn, London, WC1.	
Women's Royal Voluntary Service, 17 Old Park Lane, London, W1Y 4A	01–499–6040
Young Volunteer Force, Abbey House, 2–8, Victoria Street, London, SW1.	01–799–6043
Zimmer Orthopaedic Ltd, 134 Brompton Road, London, SW3.	01-584-6461
Bridgend, Glamorgan.	0042–3908

2 Voluntary organizations operating in England, Wales, and N. Ireland

a General

British Council for the Rehabilitation of the Disabled, Tavistock House (South), Tavistock Square, London, WC1.	01–387–4037
British Red Cross Society, 14 Grosvenor Crescent, London, SW1. Numerous local branches all over the UK.	01–235–5454
Central Council for the Disabled, 34 Eccleston Square, London, SW1.	01–834–0747
Disabled Drivers' Association, Ashwellthorpe Hall, Ashwellthorpe, Nr Norwich, NOR 89W	0508–41324
Disabled Living Foundation, Vincent House, Vincent Square, London, SW1.	01–834–8016
Disablement Income Group, Godalming, Surrey.	048–68–5181
Greater London Association for the Disabled, 183 Queensway, London, W2.	01–727–4426
Now setting up branches in local boroughs of London.	
National Fund for Research into Crippling Diseases, Vincent House, Vincent Square, London, SW1.	01–834–7001

b Specific illnesses and conditions

Arthritis and Rheumatism:	British Rheumatism and Arthritis Association, 1, Devonshire Place, London, WIN 2BD. 01–935–9905/6.
Asthma:	Asthma Research Council, 28, Norfolk Place, London, W2. (For children with asthma, contact the Invalid Children's Association, see below.)
Blind:	Royal National Institute for the Blind, 224, Great Portland Street, London, W1. 01–387–5251.
	Association for the General Welfare of the Blind, 8–22, Curtain Road, London, EC2. 01–247–2405
	Guide Dogs for the Blind, 83–89, Uxbridge Road, Ealing, London, W5. 01–567–7001.

Deaf:	Royal National Institute for the Deaf, 105, Gower Street, London, WC1. 01–387–8033. (For deaf children, see Nat. Deaf Children's Society, below.)
Deaf and Dumb:	Royal Association in aid of the Deaf & Dumb, 7, Armstrong Road, London, W3. 01–743–6187.
Diabetes:	British Diabetic Association, 3–6, Alfred Place, London, WC1. 01–636–7355.
Epilepsy:	British Epilepsy Association, 3–6, Alfred Place, London, WC1. 01–580–2704.
Haemophilia:	Haemophilia Society, 16, Trinity Street, London, SE1. 01–407–1010.
Heart:	British Heart Foundation Appeal, 57, Gloucester Place, London, W1. 01–935–0185.
Leukaemia:	Leukaemia Society, 15, Grange Road, Alvaston, Derby.
Multiple Sclerosis:	Multiple Sclerosis Society, 4, Tachbrook Street, London, SW1. 01–834–8231.
Muscular Dystrophy:	Muscular Dystrophy Group of Great Britain, 26, Borough High Street, London, SE1. 01–407–5116.
Polio:	British Polio Fellowship, Clifton House, 83/117, Euston Road, London, NW1, 01–387–5851.
Spastics:	The Spastics Society, 12, Park Crescent, London, W1. 01–636–5020.
Spina Bifida:	Association for Spina Bifida and Hydracephalus Ltd.. 112 City Road, London EC1.

c **For specific age-groups:**

I. *Children.*

National Association for Deaf, Blind and Rubella Children,
61, Senneleys Park Road, Northfield, Birmingham 31.
021–475–1392.

National Deaf Children's Society,
31, Gloucester Place, Hendon, W1.
01–486–3251/2.

Lady Hoare's Thalidomide Appeal,
78, Hamilton Terrace, London, NW8.
01–289–0231.
Cystic Fibrosis Research Trust,
Stuart House, 1, Tudor Street, London, EC4.
01–583–0989.
Invalid Children's Aid Association,
126, Buckingham Palace Road, London, SW1.
01–730–9891.

II. *Old People.*
National Old People's Welfare Council,
26, Bedford Square, London, WC1.
01–636–4066.

3 Voluntary organizations operating in Scotland

British Red Cross Society,
Alexandra House.
204, Bath Street, Glasgow, C2.
Disabled Drivers' Association,
513, Alexandra Parade, Glasgow, E1.
Disablement Income Group,
3, Howe Street, Edinburgh, 3.
Scottish Council of Social Service,
Claremont House,
18/19, Claremont Crescent, Edinburgh EH7 4HX.

Specific illnesses and conditions

Blind:	Scottish National Federation for the Welfare of the Blind, 39, St Andrew's Street, Dundee.
Deaf:	Scottish Association for the Deaf, 158, West Regent Street, Glasgow, C2.
Epilepsy:	Scottish Epilepsy Association, 24, St Vincent Place, Glasgow, C1.
Haemophilia:	Haemophilia Society, Scottish Group, 14, Orchard Drive, Edinburgh, EH4 2DY.
Heart:	Chest and Heart Association – Scottish Branch, 65, North Castle Street, Edinburgh, EH2 3LT.
Multiple Sclerosis:	Association of Scottish Branches of the Multiple Sclerosis Society, 27, Castle Street, Edinburgh, EH2 3HT.
Paraplegic:	Scottish Paraplegic (Spinal Injury) Association, 28, Gamekeepers' Road, Edinburgh, 4.

Polio: Scottish Regional Office of the British Polio Fellowship, 7, South East Circus Place, Edinburgh 3.

Spastics: Scottish Council for the Care of Spastics, 'Rhuemore', 22, Corstorphone Road, Edinburgh, 12.

Spina Bifida: Spina Bifida Association, Scotland, 24, George Square, Edinburgh 8.

Thalidomide: Lady Hoare Thalidomine Fund, Scottish Branch, 42, Orchard Road, Edinburgh 4.

4 Organizations concerned with the physically disabled in Australia

Arthritis: Australian Council for Rehabilitation of the Disabled, The White House, 403-411, George Street, Sydney, NSW.

Blind: Association of Blind Citizens of New South Wales, 44, Railway Parade Bur., Sydney.

Blind Institute (Royal Victorian), 557, St. Kilda Road, Melbourne.

Cystic Fibrosis: Australian Cystic Fibrosis Association, GPO Box 368E, Brisbane, Queensland.

Cystic Fibrosis Association of New South Wales, 60, Plateau Road, Springwood, New South Wales.

Deaf: Deaf & Dumb Society, 5, Elizabeth, Sydney.

Disabled: Foundation for the Disabled, 41, Belmore, Surrey Heights, Sydney.

Wheelchair and Disabled Association of Australia, 49, Blackbutts Road, Blrse, Sydney.

Civilian Maimed and Limbless Association, 61, Grose Camperdown, Sydney.

Epilepsy: Epileptic Welfare Association, 158, Pacific Highway North, Sydney.

Epilepsy:	Victorian Bureau for Epilepsy, 106, Wellington Parade, E, Melbourne.
Haemophilia:	Haemophilia Society, 11, Mayfield Avenue, Malvern, Melbourne.
Heart:	National Heart Foundation of Australia. Box 691, Canberra City, ACT Australia.
Multiple Sclerosis:	Australian Multiple Sclerosis Society, 13, Lytton Street, Cammeray, NSW.
Muscular Dystrophy:	Muscular Dystrophy Association of S. Australia, Inc, Pennys Hill Road, Hackham, S. Australia.
	Muscular Dystrophy Research Association of W. Australia, Inc., Box M 947 GPO, Perth, W. A. 6001.
	The New South Wales Society for Crippled Children, PO Box M10, Sydney Mail Exchange, 2012.
Paraplegic:	Paraplegic Association of New South Wales, 833, King George's Road, South Hrstvle, Sydney.
Spastics:	Australian Cerebral Palsy Association, 40, Rookwood Street, Mount Lawley, Perth, W. Australia.
Thalidomide:	Thalidomide & Amputee Children's Society, 26, Bimbadeen Cr Frnchs Frst, Sydney.
Transport for the Disabled:	Disabilities Unlimited, Lidcombe Hospital, Joseph Street, Lidcombe, Sydney.

5 Organizations concerned with the physically disabled in Canada

Arthritis & Rheumatism:	Canadian Arthritis and Rheumatism Society, 45, Charles Street, East, Toronto 5, Ontario.

Blind:	Association Canadienne Française des Aveugles, 900, Beaubien, East, Montreal, P.Q.
	Canadian Council of the Blind, 96, Ridout Street, South, London, Ontario.
	Canadian Federation of the Blind, Inc., 1172, St Mathew Street, Montreal, P.Q.
	Canadian National Institute for the Blind, Bakerwood, 1929, Bayview Avenue, Toronto 17, Ontario.
Cystic Fibrosis:	Canadian Cystic Fibrosis Federation, 51, Eglinton Avenue, East, Ste 401, Toronto 12, Ontario.
Deaf:	Canadian Association of the Deaf Inc., 485, McDonnel Street, Peterborough, Ontario.
	The Canadian Hearing Society, 60, Bedford Road, Toronto 5, Ontario.
	Canadian Association for the Hard of Hearing, 2911, Bayview Avenue, Apt 206L, Toronto.
Diabetes:	Canadian Diabetic Association, 1491, Young Street, Toronto 7, Ontario.
Disabled:	Canadian Rehabilitation Council for the Disabled, 165, Bloor Street, East, Toronto 5, Ontario.
Epilepsy:	Association for Epileptics of Quebec, 6161, St Denis Street, Suite 419, Montreal 10.
	British Columbia Epilepsy Society, Vancouver Neurological Center, 828, West Broadway, Vancouver 9.
	Ontario Epilepsy Association, 835, Quebec Street East, Toronto 8.
Haemophilia:	Canadian Haemophilia Society, 165, Bloor Street, East, Ste 303, Toronto 5, Ontario.

Heart:	Canadian Heart Foundation, 1130, Bay Street, Toronto 5, Ontario.
Multiple Sclerosis:	Multiple Sclerosis Society of Canada, 76, Avenue Road, Toronto 5.
Muscular Dystrophy:	Muscular Dystrophy Association of Canada, Rm. 307, 160, Bay Street, Toronto 5.
Paraplegic:	Canadian Paraplegic Association, 153, Lyndhurst Avenue, Toronto 4, Ontario.
Spastics:	Cerebral Palsy Section, Canadian Rehabilitation Council for the Disabled, 165, Bloor Street E, Suite 303, Toronto 5.
Traffic Injury:	Traffic Injury Research Foundation of Canada, 74, Stanley Avenue, Ottawa, Ontario.
Red Cross:	Canadian Red Cross Society, 95, Wellesley Street E Toronto 5, Ontario.

6 Organizations concerned with the physically disabled in New Zealand

Blind:	New Zealand Institute for the Blind, Box 9008, Newmarket, Auckland.
	Blinded Servicemen's Trust Board, 1a, Parnell Road, Auckland.
Cystic Fibrosis:	Capt. H. P. Griffiths, 33, Seacliffe Ave, Takapuna, Auckland 9.
Diabetic:	Diabetic Association of New Zealand, G.P.O. Box 3656, Wellington.
Disabled:	Disabled Citizen's Society Inc., 312, Dilworth Buildings, 5, Customs Street, Auckland.
	Child Welfare Division, Department of Education, Private Bag, Wellington.
	N.Z. Disabled Servicemen's Re-Establishment League, Inc., 407-410, Colonial Mutual Life Building, Wellington.

Epilepsy:	N.Z. Branch of the Brit. Epilepsy Association, Box 6436, Te Aro, Wellington.
Hard of Hearing:	Hard of Hearing League, Beehive Chambers, Courtenay Place, Wellington.
Muscular Dystrophy:	Muscular Dystrophy Research Group of New Zealand, P.O. Box 27156, Mount Roskill, New Zealand.
Multiple Sclerosis:	National Sclerosis Society, 6, Aplin Terrace, Ngaoi N4, Wellington.
Spastics:	Cerebral Palsy News, 2, Mount Hobson, Auckland 5.
Thalidomide and Crippled Children:	N.Z. Crippled Children's Society Inc., Box 5006, Lambton Quay, Wellington.

7 Organizations concerned with the physically disabled in South Africa

Blind:	National Council for the Blind, 221, Netherlands Bank Building, Pretoria.
Deaf:	National Council for the Deaf of South Africa, 119, De Korte Street, Braamfontein, Johannesburg.
Diabetic:	Department of Medicine, Medical School Observatory, Capetown.
Disabled:	Rehabilitation in South Africa, Private Bag 117, Pretoria.
Epilepsy:	The Epileptic Employment Association, Craighall, Johannesburg. National Epilepsy League, POB 2921, Pretoria.
Multiple Sclerosis:	National Multiple Sclerosis Society, 295, Villiers Road, Walmer, Port Elizabeth.
Muscular Dystrophy:	Muscular Dystrophy Association of South Africa, PO Box 142, Potchefstroom, Transvaal, SA.
Spastics:	Cerebral Palsy Division, National Council for the Care of Cripples, POB 10173, Johannesburg.

Index